CARDIOVASCULAR RESEARCH AND CLINCAL DEVELOPMENTS

HEART FAILURE: SYMPTOMS, CAUSES AND TREATMENT OPTIONS

MADISON S. WRIGHT
EDITOR

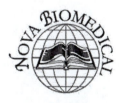

Nova Science Publishers, Inc.
New York

For permission to use material from this book please contact us:
Telephone 631-231-7269; Fax 631-231-8175
Web Site: http://www.novapublishers.com

NOTICE TO THE READER

The Publisher has taken reasonable care in the preparation of this book, but makes no expressed or implied warranty of any kind and assumes no responsibility for any errors or omissions. No liability is assumed for incidental or consequential damages in connection with or arising out of information contained in this book. The Publisher shall not be liable for any special, consequential, or exemplary damages resulting, in whole or in part, from the readers' use of, or reliance upon, this material.

Independent verification should be sought for any data, advice or recommendations contained in this book. In addition, no responsibility is assumed by the publisher for any injury and/or damage to persons or property arising from any methods, products, instructions, ideas or otherwise contained in this publication.

This publication is designed to provide accurate and authoritative information with regard to the subject matter covered herein. It is sold with the clear understanding that the Publisher is not engaged in rendering legal or any other professional services. If legal or any other expert assistance is required, the services of a competent person should be sought. FROM A DECLARATION OF PARTICIPANTS JOINTLY ADOPTED BY A COMMITTEE OF THE AMERICAN BAR ASSOCIATION AND A COMMITTEE OF PUBLISHERS.

LIBRARY OF CONGRESS CATALOGING-IN-PUBLICATION DATA
Heart failure : symptoms, causes, and treatment options / editor, Madison S. Wright.
p. ; cm.
Includes bibliographical references and index.
ISBN 978-1-61668-959-9 (hardcover)
1. Heart failure--Etiology. 2. Heart failure--Diagnosis. 3. Heart failure--Treatment. I. Wright, Madison S.
[DNLM: 1. Heart Failure--diagnosis. 2. Heart Failure--etiology. 3. Heart Failure--therapy. WG 370 H43655 2010]
RC685.C53H59 2010
616.1'29--dc22-2010014084

Published by Nova Science Publishers, Inc. ▱ *New York*

CONTENTS

PREFACE

Heart failure (HF) is a condition in which a problem with the structure or function of the heart impairs its ability to supply sufficient blood flow to meet the body's needs. This new book presents topical research in the study of heart failure including the potential use of inotropic agents in the treatment of congestive heart failure; radiation induced hazards in intervention cardiology; the utilization of different imaging methods to assess myocardial viability; the molecular mechanisms underlying the pathogenesis of heart failure; health-related quality of life issues for heart failure patients and others.

Chapter 1 - It is well known that impaired cardiac contractility is a major factor for initiating neurohormonal activation, which results in the progression and development of congestive heart failure. Since inotropic interventions improve cardiac contractility and target the core component of the pathogenesis of heart failure, these agents seem to be a good option for its treatment. The inotropes currently being used for heart failure are phosphodiesterase inhibitors, beta-adrenoceptor agonists, calcium sensitizers and cardiac glycosides. Available evidence suggests that phosphodiesterase inhibitors and beta-adrenoceptor agonists improve symptoms and hemodynamic performance in heart failure; however, these agents have been shown to increase mortality. Despite the discouraging results, these agents are still being used in the treatment of refractory heart failure with hypoperfusion or as pulse therapy in chronic end stage heart failure. On the other hand, cardiac glycosides including digoxin have beneficial effects on symptoms as well as mortality in congestive cardiac failure; however, due to low therapeutic index their serum concentration needs to be monitored carefully. Calcium sensitizers such as levosimendan, which have different mechanism of action from the traditional inotropes, show promising results in treatment of heart failure. Cardiac myosin activators, istaroxime and LASSBio 294 are newer drugs which have been reported to affect contractile function by modifying subcellular function, but their actions need to be studied in humans. Thus extensive work remains to be carried out for identifying appropriate targets for the development of inotropic agents which can be used safely for the treatment of congestive heart failure.

Chapter 2 - Heart failure (HF) is a major and growing public health problem in the United States of America (USA). Approximately 5 million patients in USA have HF, and over 550,000 new cases are diagnosed with HF each year. The current guidelines recommend cardiac catheterization to rule out Coronary Artery Disease (CAD) as the cause of newly diagnosed HF (Class I or IIa recommendation depending on the clinical scenario). Although cardiac catheterization is the gold standard in ruling out CAD, it does not provide information on viability and recovery of left ventricular function post revascularization. Determining the viability of myocardium is therefore of great clinical significance in clinical setting. Although presence of angina in patients with severe coronary vascular disease and severe left ventricular dysfunction can signify some viable myocardium, the absence of angina does not exclude the possibility of myocardial viability in similar patient population. Echocardiography and ventriculography by itself also cannot distinguish between viable and non-viable areas of myocardium as akinetic and dyskinetic areas have been seen to completely recover following revascularization. Several advanced non-invasive modalities have been developed to rule out CAD and to determine myocardial viability in patients with heart failure. The techniques most commonly used to identify viable myocardium include Thallium-201 Single-Photon Emission Computed Tomography (^{201}Tl SPECT), Technetium-99m Sestamibi imaging (Tc-99m Sestamibi), Low Dose Dobutamine Echocardiography (LDDE), Positron Emission Tomography (PET) using a combination of flow and metabolic tracer and Cardiac Magnetic Resonance imaging (CMR). Coronary Computed Tomography Angiography (CCTA) is a non invasive tool to assess coronary anatomy. The strength of CCTA lies in its very high negative predictive value; however, it does not determine the functional significance of stenosis. CCTA use in assessment of viability is currently being evaluated in multiple research studies. Extent of myocardial Thallium-201 uptake on ^{201}Tl SPECT determines the viability of myocardial tissue and thereby helps in predicting recovery post revascularization. Flouro-I8 deoxyglucose (FDG) is a metabolic tracer used in PET for determination of viability of myocardial tissue. Normal FDG uptake in areas of decreased myocardial perfusion determines the probability of myocardial recovery in those areas post revascularization. LDDE helps to determine the myocardial viability by demonstrating stress induced contractile reserve with a high specificity. This section therefore focuses on the utilization of different imaging methods to assess the myocardial viability. It also discusses the advantages and the disadvantages of different imaging techniques. The best approach depends on the individual patient and on the expertise of the reader.

Chapter 3 - Structural remodeling of the heart, including myocardial hypertrophy and fibrosis, is a key determinant for the clinical outcome of heart failure. A variety of evidence indicates the importance of neurohumoral factors, such as endothelin-1, angiotensin II, and norepinephrine for the initial phase of the development of cardiac remodeling. These agonists stimulate seven transmembrane spanning receptors that are coupled to heterotrimeric GTP-binding proteins (G proteins) of the G_i, G_q and G_{12} subfamilies. The pathophysiological roles of each G protein-mediated signaling have been revealed by studies using transgenic and knockout mice. Using specific pharmacological tools to assess the involvement of G protein signaling pathways, we have found that diacylglycerol-activated transient receptor potential canonical (TRPC) channels (TRPC3 and TRPC6), one of the downstream effectors regulated by $G\alpha_q$, work as a key mediator in the development of cardiac hypertrophy. In contrast, we also revealed that activation of $G\alpha_{12}$ family proteins in cardiomyocytes mediates pressure overload-induced cardiac fibrosis. Stimulation of purinergic $P2Y_6$ receptors by extracellular nucleotides released by mechanical stretch is a trigger of $G\alpha_{12}$-mediated fibrotic responses of the heart. Although cardiac fibrosis is believed to accompany with $G\alpha_q$-mediated pathological hypertrophy that eventually results in heart failure, our results clearly show that cardiac fibrosis and hypertrophy are independent processes. These findings will provide a new insight into the molecular mechanisms underlying pathogenesis of heart failure.

Chapter 4 - Urotensin II (UII) has been shown to cause an endothelium dependant vascular response which has been linked to hypertension and atherosclerosis. It is believed that UII acts on receptors on the intact endothelium to release NO and other vasoactive molecules to cause dilation. In individuals with a damaged endothelium it appears that UII acts directly on VSMC to cause increased contraction via the PKC pathway. More recently UII has been implicated in congestive heart failure, playing a role in cardiac contraction, hypertrophy and collagen deposition. Initial studies in animal models show that the use of UII-antagonists ameliorate the negative responses that occur following damage to the heart, further implicating UII as an important mediator of cardiac change and potential therapeutic target.

Chapter 5 - Heart failure (HF) is an escalating health problem around the world. Although recent advances in therapy for HF have improved functional capacity and survival, it is becoming increasingly clear that, for many HF patients, improving their quality of life is at least as important as the benefit that a pharmacological treatment may provide with respect to mortality.

Health-related quality of life (HRQL) is a multidimensional concept based on patients own perception of how physical, emotional and social well-being are affected by a disease or its treatment. Studies indicate that HF leads to significant impairment in all aspects of HRQL and that patients with HF have worse HRQL than the general population and patients with other chronic diseases. A worse HRQL in patients with HF has also been associated with hospital readmission and death suggesting that HRQL questionnaires could be a helpful tool to identify patients who are at increased risk of hospital readmission.

However, most published data on HRQL have been obtained from selected, hospital-based patients participating in trials. It is not known how representative they are of patients in the community. Few studies have reported the impact of HF on HRQL in the community, and there is still much less information about the comparison of HRQL in HF patients attended in different health care settings.

Recently, the INCA study evaluated HRQL in unselected outpatients in two different health care levels, Primary Care (PC) and Cardiology outpatient clinics, in Spain. Results of this study have shown that all domains of HRQL were significantly impaired in HF outpatients, and that HRQL (using the EuroQol-5D) was worse in patients with HF than in patients with other chronic diseases such as rheumatoid arthritis or type 2 diabetes, being only comparable to very severe chronic obstructive pulmonary disease. HRQL scores were worse in patients followed in PC than in Cardiology, but differences found could possibly be attributed to a large extent to the different clinical characteristics of the patients attended in each clinical setting. In spite of the differences between EuroQol-5D and Minnesota Living With Heart Failure Questionnaire, the INCA study results suggest that both questionnaires adequately reflect the severity of the disease.

Although the most original feature of the INCA study was the evaluation of HRQL in a presumably representative sample of stable HF attended in two health care settings all over a country, its results agree with the few descriptive data available in outpatients with HF.

These findings emphasize the need for a better knowledge of HRQL in HF in unselected populations, particularly about: 1) The character of its impairment in clinical subgroups; 2) Its association with the patterns of care; 3) Its prognostic meaning and its therapeutic implications; 4) Its implications for public health in the context of chronic diseases.

Chapter 6 - The advanced research in the field of biomedical nanotechnologies is concentrating on the following directions: fundamental studies of principles for the formation and function of biological nanodimensional systems; application of the acquired knowledge to the design of novel bionanomaterials, bionanotechnological processes and bionanodimensional devices; as well as particular technologies for local selective diagnostics, therapy, surgery, gene engineering and biotechnology. The enormous activity in these fields is connected with the recent achievements in cell biochemistry and molecular biology, as well as with the development of powerful physical-chemical methods and equipment. Our research is concentrating on the design of nanomaterials for the sensoring system of a biomedical robot. This robot will operate in the blood vessels (such as arteries and veins) for local selective diagnostics and treatment of venous and arterial thrombosis.

Chapter 7 - Heart failure is a major and growing public health problem in the United States as well as in the whole world. With increasing morbidity and mortality, it is primarily developed in the elderly population. The cost for the diagnosis and treatment of heart failure cause a heavy burden to the whole society.

It is crucial for a medical professional to critically evaluate diagnostic methods and therapies during the detection, management and prevention of heart failure. Heart failure is a progressive cardiac disorder. Diagnosis and appropriate treatment of heart failure at Stage A and stage B can prevent the advance to the next Stage C and Stage D. It is recognized that at stage C or Stage D, even NYHA functional class varies in response to therapy or to the progression of disease, it is impossible for a patient to reverse to Stage B. Emphasis on prevention of heart failure from stage A & B to Stage C & D is therefore utmost important.

Chapter 8 - Although there has been significant recent progress in the management of heart failure its associated mortality remains high. A large proportion of these patients die suddenly, termed sudden cardiac death (SCD), mostly from potentially reversible malignant cardiac arrhythmias. Despite the availability of a highly effective treatment in the form of an implantable cardioverter defibrillator (ICD), SCD in the heart failure population is still a significant problem. One important reason for this is the difficulty in identifying which patients are at highest risk of SCD and would benefit from an ICD. A number of tests are currently available to risk stratify heart failure patients at risk of SCD. However, used alone or in combination these are not sufficiently accurate and there is significant need for better risk stratification tools.

Multiple studies have demonstrated that serum biomarkers can accurately predict adverse outcomes in patients with heart failure of both ischaemic and non-ischaemic aetiology. A range of biomarkers predict both the occurrence of SCD in patients without ICDs and the occurrence of malignant arrhythmias in patients with devices, and in these studies individual biomarkers are at least as accurate as the current best markers of SCD risk. The pathophysiology of SCD is a complex process with a range of electrophysiological and molecular alterations contributing to arrhythmogenesis in the failing heart. By providing an assessment of these various processes, serum biomarkers may improve prediction of SCD in heart failure and help guide ICD use. Furthermore, it is likely that optimal SCD risk stratification will require the combination of multiple tests that reflect these diverse upstream processes. As such the greatest potential benefit of biomarkers may be in measuring multiple complementary markers that assess distinct aspects of arrhythmic risk.

Chapter 9 - The techniques and reproducibility of surgical coronary revascularization rely on over forty-year experience. However, surgery for ischemic heart disease with associated left ventricular dysfunction carried high if not prohibitive operative risk during the pioneering and early era of coronary surgery. Although the benefits of revascularization in this context have been well documented, the propensity to operate on patients with heart failure still often relies on concurrent anginal symptoms. Similarly, many surgeons are reluctant to offer surgery aimed to reverse low cardiac output during acute or evolving myocardial infarction.

The purpose of this chapter is to depict up-to-date strategies and attitudes toward coronary operations in chronic or acute heart failure, focusing on personal experience with ischemic cardiomyopathy and acute coronary syndromes complicated by pump dysfunction or shock. Emphasis will be given to the selection of patients, evolving technology, technical strategies, and ultimately to the limitations of isolated coronary revascularization and the increasing role of associated surgical procedures in ischemic cardiomyopathy.

In: Heart Failure: Symptoms, Causes...   ISBN: 978-1-61668-959-9
Editor: Madison S. Wright, pp. 1-28   © 2010 Nova Science Publishers, Inc.

Chapter 1

POTENTIAL USE OF INOTROPIC AGENTS IN THE TREATMENT OF CONGESTIVE HEART FAILURE

*Navneet S. Rehsia and Naranjan S. Dhalla**

Institute of Cardiovascular Sciences, St Boniface General Hospital,
Research Centre,
and Department of Physiology, Faculty of Medicine, University of
Manitoba,
Winnipeg, Canada

ABSTRACT

It is well known that impaired cardiac contractility is a major factor for initiating neurohormonal activation, which results in the progression and development of congestive heart failure. Since inotropic interventions improve cardiac contractility and target the core component of the pathogenesis of heart failure, these agents seem to be a good option for its treatment. The inotropes currently being used for heart failure are phosphodiesterase inhibitors, beta-adrenoceptor agonists, calcium sensitizers and cardiac glycosides. Available evidence suggests that

* Corresponding author: Institute of Cardiovascular Sciences, St. Boniface General Hospital Research Centre, 351 Tache Avenue, Winnipeg, Manitoba, Canada R2H 2A6, Tel: (204) 235-3417, Fax: (204) 237-0347, E-mail: nsdhalla@sbrc.ca

phosphodiesterase inhibitors and beta-adrenoceptor agonists improve symptoms and hemodynamic performance in heart failure; however, these agents have been shown to increase mortality. Despite the discouraging results, these agents are still being used in the treatment of refractory heart failure with hypoperfusion or as pulse therapy in chronic end stage heart failure. On the other hand, cardiac glycosides including digoxin have beneficial effects on symptoms as well as mortality in congestive cardiac failure; however, due to low therapeutic index their serum concentration needs to be monitored carefully. Calcium sensitizers such as levosimendan, which have different mechanism of action from the traditional inotropes, show promising results in treatment of heart failure. Cardiac myosin activators, istaroxime and LASSBio 294 are newer drugs which have been reported to affect contractile function by modifying subcellular function, but their actions need to be studied in humans. Thus extensive work remains to be carried out for identifying appropriate targets for the development of inotropic agents which can be used safely for the treatment of congestive heart failure.

1. INTRODUCTION

Cardiovascular disease has been the number one cause of mortality in adults in the past century [1]. With advent of new treatment modalities and ambulatory care for acute ischemic events like myocardial infarction and stroke, death of patients with such abnormalities has decreased by about 50% over the last decade [2]; however, there is an alarming rise in the prevalence as well as morbidity and mortality associated with congestive heart failure [1]. It is estimated that over 5 million patients in the United States of America have heart failure, and about 550 000 new patients are diagnosed each year [3]. The lifetime risk for developing congestive heart failure continues to be 1 in 5 for both men and women [4]. Major therapeutic advances in the treatment of congestive heart failure in the past three decades include angiotensin converting enzyme (ACE) inhibitors, beta-adrenoceptor blockers, heart transplantations and cardiac assist devices. Despite these interventions, one-year mortality rate in patients with congestive heart failure remains about 35% [5]; among those who are discharged alive from the hospital after acute worsening of heart failure, 7% to 16% require re-hospitalization and 45% seek emergency care by 30 days [6]. Heart failure not only has high impact on the health and quality of life, but also poses an economic burden of $35 billion to $65 billion per year in the United States alone [7].

Congestive heart failure is a complex clinical syndrome caused by structural and functional impairment that affects the filling or ejection of blood from the ventricles. The essential symptoms are dyspnea and fatigue leading to limited exercise tolerance, as well as fluid retention leading to peripheral edema and pulmonary congestion. The diagnosis is made clinically on history and physical examination; there is no single diagnostic test for heart failure. Since some patients have decreased exercise tolerance but no fluid retention (congestion) whereas others have fluid retention but good exercise tolerance, the term heart failure is preferred over the term congestive heart failure [3]. It is not a static disease but a progressive disorder resulting in neurohormonal activation leading to ventricular remodeling. Concomitant coronary artery disease and valve abnormality, if present, can also aggravate the progression [8]. ACE inhibitors, beta-adrenoceptor blockers and aldosterone-antagonists are the accepted treatment modalities of heart failure which delay the progression of heart failure by blunting the effects of various neurohormones. On the other hand, diuretics reduce congestion and provide symptomatic relief. However, as of now no satisfactory intervention is available which can stop the progression of heart failure. Therefore, all patients of heart failure suffer from gradual deterioration in the systolic function over the years.

Decreased cardiac output produces hypotension and decreased end-organ perfusion resulting in poor functioning of many organs of the body. Renal dysfunction resulting from decreased perfusion is the hallmark of refractory heart failure where most of the existing treatment modalities fail. The available drugs play some role in retarding the neurohormonal activation and the progression, but fail to deliver in settings of low cardiac output with decreased organ perfusion. Inotropic agents, by increasing the cardiac output and thus perfusion to various organs including kidneys, can be useful in such advanced cases of congestive heart failure. Patients with chronic heart failure who are on cocktail of drugs with hypotensive effect might suffer from chronic low end-organ perfusion including kidneys and heart itself. Therefore, theoretically inotropic agents given intermittently or continuously for long-term in the end-stage heart failure patients should be beneficial. Moreover, as heart failure progresses, the risk of acute exacerbation increases. Deterioration in hemodynamic functioning with increase in filling pressures and decrease in cardiac output is a major cause of acute worsening of heart failure [9]. These changes can be precipitated by events like myocardial infarction, acute ischemia, arrhythmia, non-compliance to treatment, infection as well as anemia because these situations may acutely increase cardiac preload and/or afterload or decrease contractility. However, in 40% of patients admitted with worsening of congestive heart failure, no precipitating event was found, suggesting that relentless progression of heart failure led to poor functioning and acute exacerbation [10].

Before the concept of neurohormonal activation and ventricular remodeling came to light, heart failure was considered just a defect in contractility of heart. Inotropic drugs were used in an endeavor to correct this defect, but their role in treating congestive heart failure was not studied in well-designed trials and data were scant. With the better understanding of the pathophysiology of heart failure, the focus of the research shifted to neurohormones and subcellular remodeling. This resulted in ACE inhibitors, beta-adrenoceptor blockers and aldosterone antagonists being accepted as the standard treatment. Though these drugs are successful in delaying the progression of heart failure, overall prognosis continues to be poor and the majority of patients end up with advanced heart failure or acute decompensated heart failure. So, the search of new treatment for heart failure has taken us back to inotropic agents which as a class of drugs remains to be explored in this field. In the last two decades, many trials have been conducted to investigate their effects on hemodynamics, cardiac performance, symptoms and mortality. However, no clear guidelines for their use in congestive heart failure are available. In this chapter, it is intended to discuss the trials conducted on different inotropic agents in congestive heart failure and examine their potential in the treatment.

2. ADRENOCEPTOR AGONISTS

The positive inotropic action occurs through the activation of beta-adrenoceptor mediated stimulation of adenylyl cyclase, which promotes cAMP production. Protein kinase A upon activation by cAMP, increases the influx of calcium via L-type channels during systole and also enhances the calcium uptake during diastole by activating regulatory protein phospholamban in the membrane of sarcoplasmic reticulum. These events not only increase contraction and relaxation of the cardiac muscles but also increase myocardial oxygen consumption and arrhythmogenicity [11]. Although beta-adrenoceptor mediated signal transduction mechanisms are defective in the failing heart [2, 3], various beta-adrenoceptor agonists are invariably used for improving cardiac performance in congestive heart failure. The effects of some of these agents are discussed below:

Dobutamine: At low doses, this agent increases contractility of the heart by stimulating beta-1 adrenoceptors and causes vasodilation through beta-2 adrenoceptors. At high doses, alpha-1 receptors are also stimulated by dobutamine and this results in vasoconstriction. Preliminary evaluation of dobutamine showed an improved functional capacity of the patients with severe congestive heart failure treated on a long-term but intermittent basis [12, 13]; however, these trials included only small number of patients. The DICE multicenter trial was conducted to examine the effects of low-dose intermittent dobutamine infusion in patients with severe congestive heart failure. Patients with NYHA functional class III or IV and ejection fraction $\leq$ 30% were randomly assigned to dobutamine therapy or the standard treatment and were followed up for six months. It was observed that although low-dose intermittent treatment resulted in fewer hospitalizations, the mortality rate doubled and there was no improvement in the functional status of patients [14]. Similarly, treatment of advanced heart failure with continuous intravenous dobutamine was also investigated in a randomized international trial in which the continuous dobutamine group showed higher incidence of heart dysfunction, cardiac arrest, myocardial infarction and mortality [15]. On the other hand, in patients with end-stage heart failure awaiting transplantation, continuous dobutamine therapy improved hemodynamics and decreased the number of hospitalizations [16]. In a retrospective study on 329 patients admitted with exacerbation of chronic heart failure, the effects of dobutamine therapy were compared with that of milrinone, a different type of inotropic agent. It was found that there was no difference between the two groups in terms of mortality or the clinical outcome as well as relief of symptoms; however the cost of treatment was less with dobutamine [17]. The beneficial hemodynamic effects of dobutamine on systolic heart failure were blunted if the patients were on beta-adrenoceptor blockers [18].

Xamoterol: It is a beta 1-adrenoceptor partial agonist and produces moderate increase in myocardial contractility and lowers left ventricular filling pressure at rest as well as during moderate exercise. This agent has negative chronotropic action in high sympathetic states such as strenuous exercise and treatment of patients with mild to moderate chronic heart failure showed improvement in exercise capacity and symptoms [19]. But xamoterol treatment in patients with severe heart failure showed negative inotropic and chronotropic effects [20]. A large double-blind placebo controlled study revealed that treatment of patients with xamoterol improved dyspnea but increased risk of death by 2.5-fold [21].

Ibopamine: It is an oral dopaminergic agonist which has inotropic action as well as peripheral and renal vasodilator action. Initial reports showed an improvement in the symptoms of heart failure [22, 23] but larger studies conducted later documented an increase risk of mortality with ibopamine treatment in patients with advanced heart failure [24, 25].

The existing evidence suggests that adrenergic agonists increase mortality in heart failure which can be explained by the fact that they improve contractility of heart at the expense of increasing myocardial oxygen demand. Theoretically, this could be offset by improvement in coronary perfusion by these agents [26]; however, chronically elevated catecholamines [27] and their oxidized product, adrenolutin is associated with poor prognosis of heart failure patients [28]. Furthermore, chronic exposure to catecholamines has been shown to result in cardiac apoptosis [29] and it is well-known that treatment of congestive heart failure patients with beta-adrenoceptor blockers results in decreased mortality [3]. Accordingly, neither intravenous nor long-term infusion of adrenergic agonists should be recommended. The use of beta-adrenoceptor agonists is indicated only in select patients with end-stage heart failure who will die of shock and poor perfusion if denied inotropic support. These agents can also be used in advanced heart failure patients who cannot perform activities of daily living without inotropic support. Another indication for the use of beta-adrenoceptor agonists is as a bridge to more definitive therapy such as cardiac transplantation. It should also be kept in mind that effects of these inotropic agents are blunted by prior beta-adrenoceptor blocker therapy.

3. PHOSPHODIESTERASE INHIBITORS IN CONGESTIVE HEART FAILURE

Phosphodiesterases (PDE) are intracellular enzymes which hydrolyze phosphodiester bond in cAMP and cGMP, converting them to AMP and GMP, respectively [30]. Eleven families of these enzymes have been identified and are designated as PDE1 to11. These differ in their affinities for cAMP and cGMP; PDE4 is cAMP-specific, PDE5 is cGMP-specific while PDE1 and PDE2 have comparable affinity for both cAMP and cGMP. PDE3 is unusual in its action as it has a very high affinity for both cAMP and cGMP, but its turnover rate for cAMP is much higher as compared to its turnover rate for cGMP. The individual isoforms of phosphodiesterase are localized to spatially and functionally distinct intracellular compartments in cardiomyocytes and vascular smooth muscle cells, and regulate cAMP mediated signals in these compartments [30]. Since deficient production of cAMP is one of the defects causing systolic dysfunction in patients with end-stage heart failure [31], PDE3 inhibitors have been shown to exert favorable effects on cardiac hemodynamics by increasing cAMP concentrations [32]. It was reported that milrinone a PDE3 inhibitor, increases heart rate, stroke volume, dP/dt and decreases systemic vascular resistance in heart failure patients in a dose-related manner [33].This led to numerous trials of the following PDE3 inhibitors in congestive heart failure focusing on the clinical outcomes like mortality, morbidity and length of stay in hospital:

Enoximone: In a multicentre trial including 102 patients, effects of enoximone treatment were compared with that of placebo in patients with moderate to moderately severe congestive heart failure; these patients were already being treated with conventional therapy including diuretics and digoxin. It was observed that the enoximone treated patients had higher mortality and more adverse effects than the placebo group [34]; however at low doses, enoximone showed improvement in the exercise capacity of patients with chronic heart failure [35]. Therefore a large study was planned to examine the effects of low doses of enoximone on symptoms and major clinical outcomes in patients with advanced heart failure. The Studies of Oral Enoximone Therapy in Advanced Heart Failure (ESSENTIAL) programme consisted of randomized, double-blind, placebo-controlled trials in America and Europe. The inclusion criterion for the study were ejection fraction of 30% or less, New York Heart Association class III-IV heart failure symptoms, and one hospitalization or two ambulatory visits for worsening heart failure in the previous year. The follow up period ranged from 2 months to 34 months and the median follow up duration was 16.6 months. The results showed no difference in the mortality rates and the number of cardiovascular hospitalizations; the drug had no significant adverse effects and there was no improvement in the symptoms [36]. However, oral enoximone at low doses was found to be a useful agent to wean patients with advanced heart failure from intravenous inotropic support [37].

Milrinone: The Prospective Randomized Milrinone Survival Evaluation (PROMISE) study randomly assigned 1088 patients with severe congestive heart failure with 40 mg oral milrinone per day or placebo [38]. These patients were continued on the conventional treatment including ACE inhibitor, digoxin and diuretics. After six months of treatment it was observed that milrinone therapy was associated with a 28% increase in mortality. It was also seen that patients treated with milrinone had higher rate of hospitalizations [38]. Another study, "The Outcomes of a Prospective Trial of Intravenous Milrinone for Exacerbation of Chronic Heart Failure" (OPTIME-CHF) was carried out to investigate the interaction between etiology of heart failure and response to milrinone in decompensated heart failure [39]. In this study 949 patients with systolic dysfunction and decompensated heart failure were randomized to get 48 to 72 hours of intravenous milrinone therapy or placebo. It was observed that milrinone treatment had better outcome than placebo in terms of mortality and rehospitalization in non-ischemic heart failure patients but treatment of ischemic heart failure patients with milrinone resulted in increase in mortality and rehospitalization [39]. A double-blind placebo controlled study also compared the effects of milrinone, dobutamine and placebo [40]. It was observed that inotropic therapy was safe and effective in symptomatic improvement of heart failure patients and reduced the need for hospitalizations; milrinone produced these benefits sooner than dobutamine [40].The role of combined therapy with beta-blockers and milrinone in advanced congestive heart failure has also been investigated. Hemodynamic and clinical outcomes of 65 patients with severe congestive heart failure on long-term combined treatment with milrinone and beta-blockers were examined retrospectively [41]. It was seen that there was improvement in the functional status of the patients and treatment related sudden death was relatively infrequent [41]. In another subset of patients with advanced heart failure on list for cardiac transplant, intravenous milrinone administered at home was found to be safe when used in patients with an implantable cardioverter-defibrillator [42].

Vesnarinone: Preliminary reports with fewer patients showed beneficial results with vesnarinone. In a study, patients with ejection fraction of 30% or less who were on treatment with digoxin and ACE inhibitors were randomly assigned to double-blinded therapy of 60 mg and 120 mg vesnarinone per day or placebo [43]. It was observed that with 60 mg of vesnarinone therapy for six months, there was 50% reduction in the mortality and significant improvement in the quality of life. However, 120 mg of vesnarinone was associated with higher mortality [43] but a subsequent larger study failed to demonstrate the beneficial effects of vesnarinone. Effects of vesnarinone 30 mg, 60 mg per day were compared with placebo after 9 months of treatment. It was observed that the quality of life improved with 60 mg of vesnarinone per day at 8 weeks and 16 weeks of treatment; however, the mortality rates showed a dose-dependent increase in the vesnarinone treated groups [44].

From the above data, it is evident that phosphodiesterase inhibitors differ in their clinical profile. Enoximone is associated with increased mortality at the dose which produces beneficial effects in heart failure. At low dose it has no effect on mortality but produces no improvement in symptoms as well. On the other hand, vesnarinone improved quality of life in patients with congestive heart failure but is associated with increase mortality. Similarly, milrinone is also associated with increased mortality in patients with chronic heart failure. However, it was also documented that milrinone has beneficial effects in non-ischemic heart failure. Moreover, the action of PDE inhibitor is not mediated by beta-adrenergic mechanisms because it is not attenuated by beta-adrenoceptor blockers. In fact combination of milrinone and beta-adrenoceptor blocker is considered in patients with ischemic heart failure and in patients at risk of arrhythmias. In end-stage heart failure patients with implantable cardioverter this agent has been proven to be useful. But still a lot of work is to be carried out before clear guidelines regarding the dose and length of treatment as well as selection criteria for patients are formulated. Keeping in view the high mortality associated with PDE inhibitors, these agents cannot be recommended as standard therapy as of now. Another possible use of milrinone could be as a bridge to cardiac transplantation as it is associated with more stable clinical course and less chances of developing tolerance than dobutamine [45].

4. Cardiac Glycosides

Although several cardiac glycosides have been used for the treatment of heart failure, digoxin is the most prominent agent which is still indicated for the therapy. Digoxin acts by inhibiting the Na-K ATPase pump and results in increased intracellular sodium which is then exchanged with calcium; the net increase in intracellular calcium concentration is responsible for the inotropic action. This agent improves the performance of the heart and unlike other inotropes; it does not affect the blood pressure or induce tachycardia. However, digoxin has been reported to suppress both the sympathetic drive and renin-angiotensin-aldosterone system and thus has favourable effects on neurohormonal activation [46]. The Digitalis Investigation Group (DIG) examined the effects of digoxin on mortality and morbidity in patients with heart failure in a large, double-blinded randomized trial [47]. In this trial 3397 patients with ejection fraction of $\leq 40\%$ were assigned to digoxin and 3403 patients were given placebo. Diuretics and ACE inhibitors were continued in both groups. There was no difference between the two groups in terms of rates of mortality but less number of deaths were attributed to worsening heart failure in digoxin group. Patients in digoxin group had few hospitalizations as compared to the placebo group. In an ancillary trial about 1000 patients with ejection fraction > 45% were randomly assigned to digoxin or placebo. The findings of the ancillary trial simulated the results of the main trial [47].

In another study, the effects of digoxin withdrawal were examined in patients with mild to moderate congestive heart failure [48]. Patients with chronic stable, mild to moderate congestive heart failure with systolic dysfunction without arrhythmias and on long-term treatment with diuretics and digoxin were included in the study. The results showed that the patients withdrawn from digoxin had increased incidence of failure. Patients continued on digoxin had a higher ejection fraction, lower weight and heart rate as compared to the other group [48]. A similar study was planned to investigate whether digoxin has a role when patients are receiving ACE inhibitors. A total of 178 patients with NYHA class II or III heart failure and ejection fraction $\leq$ 35% on digoxin, diuretics and ACE inhibitors were taken up for the study. Patients were randomly assigned either to continue digoxin or to be switched to placebo for twelve weeks. It was seen that withdrawal of digoxin from the patients resulted in lower quality of life scores, decreased ejection fraction, increased body weight and worsening of heart failure [49]. A subsequent analysis of these studies also made it clear that even low concentration of digoxin was sufficient to produce beneficial effects in heat failure [50]. A post-hoc analysis of DIG trial was done to investigate the association of serum digoxin concentration with mortality and hospitalization in patients with heart failure. The findings demonstrated that patients with low concentration (0.5 to 0.8 ng/ml) had a 6.3% lower mortality as compared to patients receiving placebo. Higher serum digoxin concentrations were associated with increased rate of mortality [51]. A different post-hoc analysis of the DIG trial concluded that the effect of digoxin therapy differs between men and women. In females with heart failure, digoxin therapy was associated with increased rate of mortality but no significant effect was seen in males [52]. However, analysis of the same data showed that if the serum concentration of digoxin in female patients was maintained between 0.5 and 0.9 ng/ml, it had beneficial effects on morbidity and caused no increase in mortality. At serum concentrations more than 1 ng/ml, digoxin was associated with higher risk of mortality in female patients [53]. There were concerns regarding safety of digoxin in elderly patients and risk of digoxin intoxication especially in patients with reduced renal function and low lean body mass. However, it has been documented that digoxin therapy reduces deaths and hospitalizations in patients of heart failure regardless of the age group [54]. But in patients with myocardial infarction, digoxin treatment has been associated with increase in mortality [55]. Although, in DIG trial digoxin treatment produced beneficial effects in both ischemic and non-ischemic heart failure; it failed to investigate its effects in the event of acute coronary syndromes. Therefore it should be avoided in acute myocardial infarction and in patients with persisting ischemia [55].

From the various trials, it is evident that digoxin is helpful in improving the symptoms of heart failure as well as quality of life of such patients. Though the DIG trial showed no effect on mortality of patients, the post-hoc analysis of the same study revealed that low serum digoxin concentrations were associated with reduction in mortality. As the result of these studies, digoxin is recommended as a standard therapy in moderate heart failure, it was approved by Food and Drug Administration (FDA) in 1998. The American Heart Association (AHA) recommended digoxin in patients with persistent symptoms of heart failure on diuretics, ACE inhibitors and beta-blocker therapy [3]. It should also be pointed out that for obtaining maximal benefits in terms of mortality, the serum concentration of digoxin should be maintained between 0.5 to 1.0 ng/ml [3, 51]. It is also recommended that digoxin be used with caution or avoided in post-myocardial infarction patients with persistent ischemia [3].

5. CALCIUM SENSITIZERS

In order to augment the depressed contractile force in the failing heart, a new class of drugs namely calcium sensitizers was developed [56]. These compounds not only sensitize cardiac myofilaments to the calcium ion but also inhibit PDE3 to some extent. The increased sensitivity to calcium by these agents occurs because these drugs induce changes in calcium binding to troponin C and actin-myosin complex. Although free cytoplasmic calcium released from the sarcoplasmic reticulum is responsible for increased contractility of the heart, there is no net increase in the intracellular calcium concentration, and therefore no adverse effects of calcium overload as seen with beta-agonists and PDE inhibitors. The major drugs included in this group are levosimendan and pimobendan:

Levosimendan: This agent is not only the most potent but also has a quick onset of action. It acts as calcium sensitizer at therapeutic concentrations and inhibits PDE3 at higher concentrations only [56]. Other calcium sensitizers, especially pimobendan and EMD 53998 inhibit PDE3 even at therapeutic doses. Moreover levosimendan does not impair the relaxation phase of cardiac contraction [56] and also produces vasodilatation by opening ATP-dependent K-channels in the vasculature [57]. Activation of mitochondrial ATP-sensitive K-channels results in reduction of ischemia-reperfusion injury and prevention of apoptosis [57-59]. The major advantage with levosimendan is that it improves cardiac performance without increasing myocardial oxygen consumption [60]. In patients with congestive heart failure, intravenous levosimendan treatment produced 15% or more increase in stroke volume and 25% or more decrease in pulmonary capillary wedge pressure (PCWP) in 50% patients at low dose and 88% patients at high doses. At high doses this drug caused hypotension in 5% cases and headache and nausea in less than 10% [61]. Therefore it is evident that though levosimendan is effective at low doses, it is well tolerated even at higher doses.

A large, randomized, double-blind trial including 504 patients was conducted to evaluate the safety and efficacy of levosimendan in patients with heart failure due to acute myocardial infarction (RUSSLAN Study). Levosimendan at doses of 0.1-0.4 μg/kg/min or placebo was administered intravenously for six hours [62]. Patients were observed for signs of myocardial ischemia, hypotension and worsening of heart failure. The overall mortality in both groups was also recorded. It was seen that levosimendan treatment did not cause hypotension or myocardial ischemia. However, it reduced the risk of worsening heart failure and mortality in patients with heart failure due to acute myocardial infarction. The low mortality in the levosimendan group was maintained at 180 days follow up [62]. Levosimendan was also observed to have beneficial effects on ischemia/reperfusion arrhythmia due to opening of K- ATP channels and sensitizing myocardial contractile tissue instead of increasing intracellular calcium levels during reperfusion [63]. Another study supported the use of levosimendan in short-term management of decompensated chronic heart failure. In this multicenter trial 182 patients with ejection fraction below 35% were treated with levosimendan [64]. The primary end point was hospital discharge without additional inotropic therapy and the secondary end points included changes in blood pressure, heart rate, dyspnea, pulmonary congestion and BNP. It was seen that 139 patients out of 182 responded to treatment with levosimendan and there was improvement in dyspnea and pulmonary congestion. It was also seen that there was no change in the heart rate and blood pressure [64]. In another multicenter, randomized, double-blind trial, patients with severe low-output failure were either treated with intravenous levosimendan or dobutamine [65]. The primary endpoint was hemodynamic improvement defined as an increase of 30% or more in cardiac output and a decrease of 25% or more in pulmonary-capillary wedge pressure at 24 hours of treatment. The results showed that treatment of patients with levosimendan improved hemodynamics more effectively than treatment with dobutamine. It was also observed that levosimendan was associated with lower mortality as compared to dobutamine [65].

Further understanding of the mechanism of action of levosimendan it became clear that it also has antioxidant and anti-inflammatory effects. In this regard, 25 patients suffering from decompensated heart failure on standard therapy were randomized to receive 24 hours intravenous treatment with levosimendan or dobutamine [66]. Patients were checked for their blood levels of brain natriuretic peptide (BNP), interleukin-6 (IL-6), tumor necrosis factor alpha (TNF-α) and malondialdehyde (MDA) at presentation as well as at 48 hours and 5 days post-treatment. The analysis of results revealed that levosimendan treated group had reduction in BNP as compared to baseline at both 48 hours and 5 days. IL-6 and MDA levels showed reduction at 5 days. TNF-α however did not show significant reduction. When compared to the dobutamine group, BNP and IL-6 levels were lower at 5 days in levosimendan group [66]. In a similar study, it was seen that treatment with either levosimendan or dobutamine in patients with decompensated heart failure resulted in reduction in NT-proBNP, but levosimendan had better and prolonged effects as compared to dobutamine [67]. It is thus evident that levosimendan not only improved hemodynamics but also affected neurohormonal progression and cardiac remodeling by its antioxidant and anti-inflammatory actions. However, a multicenter trial failed to demonstrate the superiority of levosimendan over dobutamine in terms of mortality and symptoms as assessed by patients. There was higher incidence of cardiac failure in dobutamine group and more adverse effects like atrial fibrillation, headache and hypokelemia in levosimendan group [68]. Most of the studies with levosimendan used an intravenous route; however oral levosimendan was tested by Cheng et al [69] in a study on mongrel dogs with pacing induced heart failure. It was observed that oral therapy with levosimendan increased contractility as well as vasodilatation in normal and heart failure dogs [69].

Pimobendan: This drug has also been studied extensively in patients with congestive heart failure. It was found to exert favorable effects on hemodynamics resulting in reduction of left ventricular end-diastolic wall stress (preload) and end-systolic wall stress (afterload). It increased stroke volume index and yet had favorable effects on myocardial oxygen consumption [70, 71]. Pimobendan was also documented to produce symptomatic relief in patients with congestive heart failure. In a multicenter trial, 198 patients with moderate to severe heart failure were randomized to four groups which would receive a daily oral dose of pimobendan 2.5 mg, 5.0 mg, 10 mg or placebo for 12 weeks [72]. The change in quality of life of patients and their ability to exercise was studied. It was found that pimobendan 5 mg daily given for 12 weeks was well tolerated and significantly increased the duration of exercise and quality of life [72]. In another study it was demonstrated that in patients with severe chronic heart failure who are not responding to the combination of digoxin, diuretics and ACE inhibitors; add-on therapy with pimobendan resulted in improvement [73]. To study the long-term effects and safety of pimobendan, treatment with this agent was compared with that using enalapril where 242 patients with mild to moderate congestive heart failure on diuretics and digitalis were randomized to receive either enalapril or pimobendan for six months. It was demonstrated that both pimobendan and enalapril were well tolerated and produced comparable improvements in exercise duration and dyspnea. Even the mortality rates were similar [74]. However, another large multicenter trial carried out to evaluate the long-term effects of pimobendan therapy showed different results. Pimobendan in Congestive Heart Failure (PICO) trial enrolled 317 patients with NYHA class II to III congestive heart failure despite ACE inhibitors and diuretics. Patients were randomized to receive either pimobendan (1.25 or 2.5 mg twice daily) or placebo for six months. It demonstrated that pimobendan treatment improved hemodynamics in congestive heart failure with no increased risk of arrhythmias. However the mortality rate was more in pimobendan group and there was no improvement in the quality of life [75].

From the above mentioned observations, it appears that calcium sensitizers, pimobendan and levosimendan, differ in their clinical profile in terms of mortality. Though the results of the clinical trials with pimobendan were encouraging, the mortality data from the PICO trial raised concerns regarding the safety of the drug. On the other hand, mortality trials with levosimendan have shown improved survivals in patients with chronic heart failure. As a result, levosimendan is now recommended by the European Society of Cardiology in patients with symptomatic low cardiac output heart failure secondary to cardiac systolic dysfunction without severe hypotension [76]. Reasons for this difference in clinical profile could be the immunomodulatory and anti-apoptotic effects of levosimendan. Moreover, pimobendan can inhibit PDE3 even at low doses while levosimendan does it only at very high doses.

6. NOVEL INOTROPES

Since contractile force development in the heart is determined by the coordination function of subcellular organelles such as sarcolemma, sarcoplasmic reticulum, myofibrils and mitochondria [77, 78] some effort is being made to target those sites for discovering new inotropic agents for the treatment of heart failure.

Cardiac myosin activators: These agents such as CK-1827452 activate myocardial myosin ATPase resulting in effective myosin cross-bridge formation and increased myocyte contractility [79]. These drugs also improve energy utilization by inhibiting non-productive consumption of ATP. Moreover, they have the advantage of not producing any effect on intracellular calcium or cAMP [79]. As the mechanism of action of myosin activators is independent of adrenergic stimulation, beta-blockers do not reverse their inotropic action. Studies using rat and dog models of heart failure showed that myosin activators improved cardiac contractility in a dose-dependent manner without changing intracellular calcium levels [80]. The first human study was done in 2006, and the aim was to determine the maximally tolerated dose, pharmacokinetics, safety and tolerability of CK-1827452, and to evaluate its effects on left ventricular systolic function. It revealed that CK-1827452 was well tolerated at dose of 0.5 mg/kg/h for 6 hours and below, but patients who received 0.75 and 1.0 mg/kg/h dose developed signs and symptoms of myocardial ischemia. It was also evident that it increased the ejection fraction and fractional shortening by a unique mechanism i.e. by directly increasing systolic ejection time rather than contraction velocity. There were no increases in adverse effects and no changes in heart rate or electrocardiographic PR and QT intervals at 0.5 mg/kg/h dose [79]. These agents are in the initial phase of the research and more work needs to be done to examine their effects on morbidity and mortality in patients with chronic heart failure.

Istaroxime (PST2744): It is a novel agent that has inotropic effects through Na-K-ATPase inhibition and lusitropic action via stimulation of the sarcoplasmic reticulum calcium ATPase isoform 2 (SERCA-2). It improves cardiac contractility as well as diastolic relaxation [81]. Preliminary studies on istaroxime treatment in acute decompensated heart failure patients have shown that it decreases pulmonary-capillary wedge pressure, improves diastolic dysfunction, increases systolic blood pressure and decreases heart rate [82]. At present there is no data about its suitability for long-term treatment in chronic heart failure and on clinical outcomes like mortality, morbidity and hospitalizations.

Flosequinan: It is an arterial and venodilator which acts by interfering with inositol-triphosphate/protein kinase pathway, but also has inotropic properties [83]. It has beneficial effects on symptoms of heart failure [84] but is accompanied by activation of sympathetic and renin-angiotensin system and increased risk of mortality [85, 86].

Table 1. Effects of different inotropic agents on mortality in congestive heart failure

Inotropic agent	Mechanism of action	Effects on mortality	Reference
Dobutamine	beta-adrenoceptor agonist	increase	Oliva F et al [14]; O'Connor CM et al [15]
Xamoterol	beta-adrenoceptor agonist	increase	Xamoterol study group [21]
Ibopamine	dopaminergic	increase	Feenstra J et al [24]; Hampton JR [25]
Enoximone	phosphodiesterase inhibitor	increase	Uretsky BF et al [34]; Metra M et al [36]
Milrinone	phosphodiesterase inhibitor	increase	Packer M et al [38]; Felker GM et al [39]
Vesnarinone	phosphodiesterase inhibitor	increase	Cohn JN et al [44]
Digoxin	Na-K-ATPase inhibitor	decrease at low serum concentration	Digitalis Investigation Group [47]; Rathore SS et al [51];

			Adams KF Jr et al [53]
Levosim endan	calcium sensitizer	decrease	Moiseyev et al [62]; Follath F et al [65]
Pimoben dan	calcium sensitizer	increase	Lubsen J et al [75]
Cardiac myosin activator	activate myocardial myosin ATPase	no data available	Teerlink JR [79]
Istaroxim e	Na-K-ATPase inhibition and SERCA-2 stimulation	no data available	Kelso EJ et al [83]
Flosequi nan	IP$_3$/Protein kinase pathway	increase	Massie BM et al [86]
LASSBi o 294	sarcoplasmic reticulum Ca^{2+}uptake/ release	no data available	Sudo RT et al [87]

LASSBio-294: It is a new compound which exerts positive inotropic action through an interaction with the Ca^{2+}-uptake/release process resulting in accumulation of Ca^{2+} into the sarcoplasmic reticulum. It has no effect on the rate and rhythm of the heart [87]. In addition it also exhibits vasodilator action through inhibition of PDE5 [88]; however, very little has been done to investigate the role of this drug in heart failure.

7. CONCLUDING REMARKS

The available treatment options for chronic heart failure have failed to prevent the progression of heart failure. These patients are prone to decompensation resulting in frequent acute exacerbations. Over the course of time, majority of the patients with chronic heart failure end up in an advanced stage with severely reduced contractility, hypotension and hypoperfusion of vital organs. The treatment at this stage is frustrating because of the lack of therapeutic options. Thus a great deal of work has been carried out for establishing inotropic agents as a new class of drugs for the treatment of heart failure [Table 1]. Inotropic agents, by acting on the core defect to improve cardiac contractility, seemed to be an attractive choice but studies done on beta-adrenoceptor agonists and phosphodiesterase inhibitors have shown increased mortality. Partly, this increase in mortality is attributed to increased oxygen consumption, arrhythmogenicity and detrimental effect such as myocardial ischemia. Though preventing death is the primary goal, improving symptoms and quality of life as well as decreasing hospitalizations and emergency visits are important secondary goals. Moreover, to avoid unintended effects of therapy, low doses which do not produce effects beyond hemodynamic improvement in carefully selected patients needs to be studied. Treatment of end-stage heart failure with hypoperfusion of vital organs is a challenge and an important issue is whether to improve the quality of life by using phosphodiesterase inhibitors or deny these agents because of risk of decreased survival. Also, there is no method to quantify the risk of death in any particular patient. Hypoperfusion of heart resulting in ischemia can start a vicious circle of myocardial injury and further depress cardiac function. On the other hand, there is risk of 'inotropic dependence' even with short-term therapy. It has been postulated that beta-adrenoceptor agonists and phosphodiesterase inhibitors increase contractility of the heart at the expense of acceleration of the underlying disease like ischemic heart disease. This can lead to deterioration in functioning of heart and inability of the heart to work without inotropic support [26]. Therefore it is evident from the available data that beta-adrenoceptor agonists and phosphodiesterase inhibitors cannot be recommended as a standard therapy in chronic heart failure as well as acute exacerbations. However, in carefully selected patients with hypotension leading to hypoperfusion and/or worsening renal function, these agents can be used as a last resort and can also be used as a "pharmacological bridge" in patients waiting for definitive therapy such as cardiac transplantation.

It is observed that digoxin is an underused drug. Although it is recommended by AHA and approved by FDA, its use is still decreasing. This may be because of the introduction of ACE inhibitors, beta-blockers and aldosterone antagonists which have a proven role in decreasing mortality. Drug interactions and concerns about increased mortality in women may also have contributed [55] but these concerns were proven false. Moreover, it does not have a hypotensive effect and it can find special use in heart failure patients with arrhythmias. Another advantage is the absence of adverse effects on electrolytes and renal functions as seen with ACE inhibitors. It has a low cost which can be an important factor in developing countries. So, digoxin is strongly recommended for patients with systolic heart failure on treatment with ACE inhibitors, beta-blockers and aldosterone antagonist. However, it should be avoided in patients with ongoing ischemia.

On the other hand, among calcium sensitizers, levosimendan seems to be a promising drug with favorable effects on symptoms, hemodynamic and mortality in patients with heart failure. Apart from inotropic action it has neurohormonal modulatory effects; however, well-designed, larger trials are needed before any guidelines can be formulated. Other inotropic agents such as Istaroxime and myosin activators are in the initial phase of research and their potential will be explored in the coming years.

ACKNOWLEDGMENTS

The work in this study was supported by a grant from the Canadian Institutes of Health Research. The infrastructure support for this project was provided by the St. Boniface General Hospital Research Foundation.

REFERENCES

[1]   Miller, L. W. & Missov, E. D. (2001). Epidemiology of heart failure. *Cardiology Clinics. 19*, 547-55.

[2]   Klein, L; O'Connor, C. M, Gattis, W. A., Zampino, M. & Gheorghiade, M. et al. (2003) . Pharmacologic therapy for patients with chronic heart failure and reduced systolic function: review of trials and practical considerations. *Am J Cardiol., 91*, 18-40.

[3]   Chin, M. H., Feldman, A. M., Francis, G. S., Konstam, M. A. & Yancy, C. W. et al. (2009). 2009 focused update incorporated into the ACC/AHA 2005 guidelines for the diagnosis and management of heart failure in adults: a report of the American College of Cardiology Foundation/American Heart Association task force on practice guidelines. *Circulation., 119*, 391-479.

[4]   Lloyd-Jones, D. M., Larson, M. G., Leip, E. P., Beiser, A. & Levy, D. et al. (2002). Lifetime risk for developing congestive heart failure: the Framingham heart study. *Circulation., 106*, 3068-72.

[5]   Zannad, F., Briancon, S., Juilliere, Y., Alla, F. & Virion, J. M. et al. (1999). Incidence, clinical and etiologic features and outcomes of advanced chronic heart failure: The EPICAL Study. *J Am Coll Cardiol., 33*, 734-42.

[6]   Ezekowitz, J. A., Bakal, J. A., Kaul, P., Westerhout, C. M. & Armstrong, P. W. (2008). Acute heart failure in the emergency department: short and long-term outcomes of elderly patients with heart failure. *Eur J Heart Fail., 10*, 308-14.

[7] Lloyd-Jones, D., Adams, R., Carnethon, M., De Simone, G. & Hong, Y. et al. (2009). Heart disease and stroke statistics—2009 update: a report from the American Heart Association Statistics Committee and Stroke Statistics Subcommitte. *Circulation., 119*, 21-181.

[8] Baig, M. K., Mahon, N., McKenna, W. J., Caforio, A. L. & Gheorghiade, M. et al. (1998). The pathophysiology of advanced heart failure. *Am Heart J., 135*, 216-30.

[9] Jain, P., Massie, B. M., Gattis, W. A., Klein, L. & Gheorghiade, M. (2003). Current medical treatment for the exacerbation of chronic heart failure resulting in hospitalization. *Am Heart J., 145*, 3-17.

[10] Opasich, C., Rapezzi, C., Lucci, D., Gorini, M. & Maggioni, A. P. et al. (2001). Precipitating factors and decision-making processes of short-term worsening heart failure despite optimal treatment. *Am J Cardiol., 88*, 382-7.

[11] Vroom, M. B. (2006). An overview of inotropic agents. *Seminars in Cardiothoracic and Vascular Anesthesia., 10*, 246-52.

[12] Roffman, D. S., Applefeld, M. M., Grove, W. R., Talesnick, B. S. & Reed, W. P. et al. (1985). Intermittent dobutamine hydrochloride infusions in outpatients with chronic congestive heart failure. *Clin Pharm., 4*, 195-9.

[13] Krell, M. J., Kline, E. M., Bates, E. R., Hodgson, J. M. & Pitt, B. et al. (1986). Intermittent, ambulatory dobutamine infusions in patients with severe congestive heart failure. *Am Heart J. 12,* 787-91.

[14] Oliva, F., Latini, R., Politi, A., Nicolas, E. & Mauri, F. et al. (1999). Intermittent 6-month low-dose dobutamine infusion in severe heart failure: DICE multicenter trial. *Am Heart J., 138,* 247-53.

[15] O'Connor, C. M., Gattis, W. A., Uretsky, B. F., Adams, K. F. & Califf, R. M. et al. (1999). Continuous intravenous dobutamine is associated with an increased risk of death in patients with advanced heart failure: insights from the Flolan International Randomized Survival Trial (FIRST). *Am Heart J., 138,* 78-86.

[16] Upadaya, S., Lee, F. A., Saldarriaga, C., Verma, S. & Katz, S. D. et al. (2004). Home continuous positive inotropic infusion as a bridge to cardiac transplantation in patients with end-stage heart failure. *J Heart Lung Transplant., 23,* 466-72.

[17] Yamani, M. H., Haji, S. A., Starling, R. C., Kelly, L. & Young, J. B. et al. (2001). Comparisons of dobuatamine-based and milrinone-based therapy for advanced decompensated congestive heart failure:

Hemodynamic efficacy, clinical outcome, and economic impact. *Am Heart J, 142,* 998-1002.

[18] Triposkiadis, F., Dalampiras, P., Kelepeshis, G., Skoularigis, J. & Sitafidis, G. (2008). Hemodynamic effects of dobutamine in patients with an exacerbation of chronic systolic heart failure treated with low doses of carvedilol. *Int J Clin Pharmacol Ther., 46,* 136-9.

[19] Furlong, R. & Brogden, R. N. (1988). Xamoterol. A preliminary review of its pharmacodynamic and pharmacokinetic properties, and therapeutic use. *Drugs., 36,* 455-74.

[20] Pouleur, H., Hanet, C. & Rousseau, M. F. (1990). Clinical experience of therapy with xamoterol in patients with severe systolic and diastolic dysfunction. *Eur Heart J., 11,* 33-8.

[21] The xamoterol in severe heart failure study group. (1990). Xamoterol in severe heart failure. *Lancet., 336,* 1-6.

[22] Arcensio, S. R., Barretto, A. C., Szambock, F., Mady, C. & Pileggi, F. et al. (1994). Comparative study between ibopamine and captopril in mild and moderate heart failure. A double-blind study. *Arq Bras Cardiol., 63,* 409-13.

[23] Barabino, A., Galbariggi, G., Pizzorni, C. & Lotti, G. (1991). Comparative effects of long-term therapy with captopril and ibopamine in chronic congestive heart failure in old patients. *Cardiology., 78,* 243-56.

[24] Feenstra, J., van der Linden, P. D., in't Veld, B. A., Grobbee, D. E. & Stricker, B. H. (1998). Risk factors for mortality in users of ibopamine. *Br J Clin Pharmacol., 46,* 71-7.

[25] Hampton, J. R., Kleber, F. X., Cowley, A. J., Ardia, A. & Skene, A. M. et al. (1997). Randomised study of effect of ibopamine on survival in patients with advanced severe heart failure. Second prospective randomized study of ibopamine on mortality and efficacy (PRIME-II) investigators. *Lancet., 349,* 971-7.

[26] Felker, G. M. & O'Connor, C. M. (2001). Inotropic therapy for heart failure: an evidence-based approach. *Am Heart J., 142,* 393-401.

[27] Cohn, J. N., Levine, T. B., Oliviari, M. T., Garberg, V. & Rector, T. et al. (1984). Plasma norepinephrine as a guide to prognosis in patients with chronic congestive heart failure. *N Eng J Med., 311,* 819-23.

[28] Rouleau, J. L., Pitt, B., Dhalla, N. S., Dhalla, K. S. & Packer, M. et al. (2003). Prognostic importance of the oxidized product of catecholamines, adrenoleutin, in patients with severe heart failure. *Am Heart J., 145,* 926-32.

[29] Colucci, W. S., Sawyer, D. B., Singh, K. & Communal, C. (2000). Adrenergic overload and apoptosis in heart failure: implications for therapy. *J Card Fail., 6,* 1-7.

[30] Movsesian, M., Stehlik, J., Vandeput, F. & Bristow, M. R. (2009). Phosphodiesterase inhibition in heart failure. *Heart Fail Rev., 14,* 255-263.

[31] Feldman, M. D., Copelas, L., Gwathmey, J. K., Phillips, P., Warren, S. E., Schoen, F. J., Grossman, W. & Morgan, J. P. (1987). Deficient production of cyclic AMP: pharmacological evidence of an important cause of contractile dysfunction in patients with end-stage heart failure. *Circulation., 75,* 331-339.

[32] Gilbert, E. M., Hershberger, R. E., Wiechmann, R. J., Movsesian, M. A. & Bristow, M. R. (1995). Pharmacologic and hemodynamic effects of combined beta-agonist stimulation and phosphodiesterase inhibition in failing human heart. *Chest., 108,* 1524-1532.

[33] Jaski, B. E., Fifer, M. A., Wright, R. F., Braunwald, E. & Colucci, W. S. (1985). Positive inotropic and vasodilator actions of milrinone in patients with severe congestive heart failure. Dose-response relationships and comparison to nitroprusside. *J Clin Invest., 75,* 643-649.

[34] Uretsky, B. F., Jessup, M., Konstam, M. A., Dec, G. W., Leier, C. V., Benotti, J., Murali, S., Herrmann, H. C. & Sandberg, J. A. (1990). Multicenter trial of oral enoxamine in patients with moderate to moderately severe congestive heart failure. Lack of benefit compared with placebo. Enoxamine Multicenter Trial Group. *Circulation., 82,* 774-780.

[35] Lowes, B. D., Higginbotham, M., Petrovich, L., DeWood, M. A. & Bristow, M. R. et al. (2000). Low-dose enoximone improves exercise capacity in chronic heart failure. Enoxamine Study Group. *J Am Coll Cardiol., 36,* 501-8.

[36] Metra, M., Eichhorn, E., Abraham, W. T., Linseman, J. & Bristow, M. R. et al. (2009). Effects of low-dose oral enoximone administration on mortality, morbidity, and exercise capacity in patients with advanced heart failure: the randomized, double-blind, placebo-controlled, parallel group ESSENTIAL trials. *Eur Hear J., 30,* 3015-26.

[37] Feldman, A. M., Oren, R. M., Abraham, W. T., Boehmer, J. P. & Bristow, M. R. et al. (2007). Low-dose oral enoximone enhances the ability to wean patients with ultra-advanced heart failure from

intravenous inotropic support: results of the oral enoximone in intravenous inotrope-dependent subjects trial. *Am Heart J., 154,* 861-9.

[38] Packer, M., Carver, J. R., Rodeheffer, R. J., Ivanhoe, R. J., DiBianco, R., Zeldis, S. M., Hendrix, G. H., Bommer, W. J., Elkayam, U. & Kukin, M. L. et al. (1991). Effect of oral milrinone on mortality in severe chronic heart failure. The PROMISE Study Research Group. *N Eng J Med., 325,* 1468-75.

[39] Felker, G. M., Benza, R. L., Chandler, A. B., Cuffe, M. S. & O'Connor, C. M. et al. (2003). Heart Failure Etiology and Response to Milrinone in Decompensated Heart Failure: Results from the OPTIME-CHF Study. *J Am Coll Cardiol., 41,* 997-1003.

[40] Lopez-Candales, A., Vora, T., Gibbons, W., Carron, C. & Schwartz, J. et al. (2002). Symptomatic improvement in patients treated with intermittent infusion of inotropes: a double-blind placebo controlled pilot study. *J Med., 33,* 129-46.

[41] Zewail, A. M., Nawar, M., Vrtovec, B., Eastwood, C. & Kar, M. N. et al. (2003). Intravenous milrinone in treatment of advanced congestive heart failure. *Tex Heart Inst J., 30,* 109-13.

[42] Brozena, S. C., Twomey, C., Goldberg, L. R., Desai, S. S. & Jessup, M. et al. (2004). A prospective study of continuous intravenous milrinone therapy for status IB patients awaiting heart transplant at home. *J Heart Lung Transplant., 23,*1082-6.

[43] Feldman, A. M., Bristow, M. R., Parmley, W. W., Carson, P. E. & Bain, R. P. et al. (1993). Effects of vesnarinone on morbidity and mortality in patients with heart failure. Vesnarinone Study Group. *N Eng J Med., 329,* 149-55.

[44] Cohn, J. N., Goldstein, S. O., Greenberg, B. H., Lorell, B. H. & White, B. G. et al. (1998). A dose-dependent increase in mortality with vesnarinone among patients with severe heart failure. Vesnarinone Trial Investigators. *N Eng J Med., 339,* 1810-6.

[45] Mehra, M. R., Ventura, H. O., Kapoor, C., Zimmerman, D. & Smart, F. W. et al. (1997). Safety and clinical utility of long-term intravenous milrinone in advanced heart failure. *Am J Cardiol., 80,* 61-4.

[46] Teerlink, J. R., Metra, M., Sabbah, H. N., Cotter, G. & Gheorghiade, M. et al. (2009). Agents with inotropic properties for the management of acute heart failure syndromes. Traditional agents and beyond. *Heart Fail Rev., 14,* 243-53.

[47] The Digitalis Investigation Group. (1997). The effect of digoxin on mortality and morbidity in patients with heart failure. *N Eng J Med., 336,* 525-33.

[48] Uretsky, B. F., Young, J. B., Shahidi, F. E., Yellen, L. G. & Jolly, M. K. et al. (1993). Randomized study assessing the effect of digoxin withdrawl in patients with mild to moderate chronic congestive heart failure: results of the PROVED trial. PROVED Investigative Group. *J Am Coll Cardiol., 22,* 955-62.

[49] Packer, M., Gheorghiade, M., Young, J. B., Adams, K. F. & Jolly, M. K. et al. (1993). Withdrawal of digoxin from patients with chronic heart failure treated with angiotensin-converting-enzyme inhibitors. RADIANCE Study. *N Eng J Med., 329,* 1-7.

[50] Adams, K. F., Gheorghiade, M., Uretsky, B. F., Patterson, J. H. & Young, J. B. et al. (2002). Clinical benefits of low serum digoxin concentrations in heart failure. *J Am Coll Cardiol., 39,* 946-53.

[51] Rathore, S. S., Curtis, J. P., Wang, Y., Bristow, M. R. & Krumholz, H. M. et al. (2003). Association of serum digoxin concentration and outcomes in patients with heart failure. *JAMA., 289,* 871-8.

[52] Rathore, S. S., Wang, Y. & Krumholz, H. M. (2002). Sex-based differences in the effect of digoxin for the treatment of heart failure. *N Eng J Med., 347.,* 1403-11.

[53] Adams, K. F. Jr, Patterson, J. H., Gattis, W. A., O'Connor, C. M., Gheorghiade, M. et al. (2005). Relationship of serum digoxin concentration to mortality and morbidity in women in the digitalis investigation group trial: a retrospective analysis. *J Am Coll Cardiol., 46,* 497-504.

[54] Rich, M. W., McSherry, J., Williford, W. O. & Yusuf, S. (2001). Effect of age on mortality, hospitalizations and response to digoxin in patients with heart failure: the DIG study. *J Am Coll Cardiol., 38,* 806-13.

[55] Gheorghiade, M., van Veldhuisen, D. J. & Colucci W. S. (2006). Contemporary use of digoxin in the management of cardiovascular disorders. *Circulation., 113,* 2556-64.

[56] Haikala, H. & Linden, I. B. (1995). Mechanisms of action of calcium-sensitizing drugs. *J Cardiovasc Pharmacol., 26,* 10-9.

[57] Lehtonen, L. A. (2001). Levosimendan: a parenteral calcium-sensitising drug with additional vasodilatory properties. *Expert Opin Investig Drugs., 10,* 955-70.

[58] Grover, G. J. & Garlid, K. D. (2000). ATP-sensitive potassium channels: a review of their cardioprotective pharmacology. *J Mol Cell Cardiol.*, *32*, 677-95.

[59] Kowaltowski, A. J., Seetharaman, S., Paucek, P. & Garlid, K. D. (2001). Bioenergetic consequences of opening the ATP-sensitive K(+) channel of heart mitochondria. *Am J Physiol Heart Circ Physiol.*, *280*, 649-57.

[60] Lilleberg, J., Nieminen, M. S., Akkila, J., Mattila, S. & Salmenpera, M. et al. (1998). Effects of a new calcium sensitizer, levosimendan, on hemodynamics, coronary blood flow and myocardial substrate utilization early after coronary artery bypass grafting. *Eur Heart J.*, *19*, 660-8.

[61] Nieminen, M. S., Akkila, J., Kleber, F. X., Lehtonen, L. A. & Remme, W. J. et al. (2000). Hemodynamic and neurohumoral effects of continuous infusion of levosimendan in patients with congestive heart failure. *J Am Coll Cardiol.*, *36*, 1903-12.

[62] Moiseyev, V. S., Ruda, M. Y., Golikov, A. P., Laine, T. & Lie, K. I. et al. (2002). Safety and efficacy of a novel calcium sensitizer, levosimendan, in patients with left ventricular failure due to an acute myocardial infarction. A randomized, placebo-controlled, double-blind study (RUSSLAN). *Eur Heart J.*, *23*, 1422-32.

[63] Du Toit, E. F., Muller, C. A., McCarthy, J. & Opie, L. H. (1999). Levosimendan: effects of calcium sensitizer on function and arrhythmias and cyclic nucleotide levels during ischemia/reperfusion in the Langendorff-perfused guinea pig heart. *J Pharmacol Exp Ther.*, *290*, 505-14.

[64] Bocchi, E. A., Vilas-Boas, F., Lage, S., Albuquerque, D. & Baima, J. et al. (2008). Levosimendan in decompensated heart failure patients: efficacy in a Brazilian cohort. Results of the BELIEF study. *Arq Bras Cardiol.*, *90*, 182-90.

[65] Follath, F., Cleland, J. G., Just, H., Papp, J. G. & Lehtonen, L. et al. (2002). Efficacy and safety of intravenous levosimendan compared with dobutamine in severe low-output heart failure (the LIDO study): a randomized double-blind trial. *Lancet.*, *360*, 196-202.

[66] Avgeropoulou, C., Andreadou, I., Demopoulou, M., Missovoulos, P., Kallikazaros, I. et al. (2005). The Ca^{2+}-sensitizer levosimendan improves oxidative damage, BNP and pro-inflammatory cytokine levels in patients with advanced decompensated heart failure in comparison to dobutamine. *Eur J Heart Fail.*, *7*, 882-7.

[67] Cavusoglu, Y., Tek, M., Birdane, A., Ata, N., Timuralp, B. et al. (2008). Both levosimendan and dobutamine treatments result in significant

reduction of NT-proBNP levels, but levosimendan has better and prolonged neurohormonal effects than dobutamine. *Int J Card., 127,* 188-191.

[68] Mebazaa, A., Nieminen, M. S., Packer, M., Kleber, F. X. & Kivikko, M. et al. (2007). Levosimendan vs dobutamine for patients with acute decompensated heart failure: the Survive randomized trial. *JAMA., 297,* 1883-91.

[69] Masutani, S., Cheng, H. J., Levijoki, J., Little, W. C. & Cheng, C. P. et al. (2008). Orally available levosimendan dose-related positive inotropic and lusitropic effect in conscious chronically instrumented normal and heart failure dogs. *J Pharmac Exp Therap., 325,* 236-47.

[70] Hasenfuss, G., Holubarsch, C., Heiss, H. W., Allgeier, M. & Just, H. (1989). Effects of pimobendan on hemodynamics and myocardial energetics in patients with idiopathic dilated cardiomyopathy: comparison with nitroprusside. *J Cardiovasc Pharmacol.,* 14., 31-5.

[71] Remme, W. J., Kruijssen, D. A., Krauss, X. H., Bartels, G. L. & de Leeuw, P. W. et al. (1994). Hemodynamic, neurohumoral, and myocardial energetic effects of pimobendan, a novel calcium-sensitizing compound, in patients with mild to moderate heart failure. *J Cardiovasc Pharmacol., 24,* 730-9.

[72] Kubo, S. H., Gollub, S., Bourge, R., Rahko, P. & Shanes, J. et al. (1992). Beneficial effects of pimobendan on exercise tolerance and quality of life in patients with heart failure. Results of a multicenter trial. The Pimobendan Multicenter Research Group. *Circulation., 85,* 942-9.

[73] Hagemeijer, F. (1991). Intractable heart failure despite angiotensin-converting enzyme inhibitors, digoxin, and diuretics: long-term effectiveness of add-on therapy with pimobendan. *Am Heart J., 122,* 517-22.

[74] Remme, W. J., Baumann, G., Frick, M. H., Haehl, M. & Baiker, W. et al. (1994). Long-term efficacy and safety of pimobendan in moderate heart failure. A double-blind parallel 6-month comparison with enalapril. The Pimobendan-Enalapril Study Group. *Eur Heart J., 15,* 947-56.

[75] Lubsen, J., Just, H., Remme, W. J., Dumont, J. M. & Seed, P. et al. (1996). Effect of pimobendan on exercise capacity in patients with heart failure: main results from the pimobendan in congestive heart failure (PICO) trial. *Heart., 76,* 223-31.

[76] Parissis, J. T., Rafouli-Stergiou, P., Paraskevaidis, I. & Mebazaa, A. (2009). Levosimendan: from basic science to clinical practice. *Heart Fail Rev., 14,* 265-75.

[77] Dhalla, N. S., Dent, M. R., Tappia, P. S., Sethi, R., Barta, J. & Goyal, R. K. (2006). Subcellular remodeling as a viable target for the treatment of congestive heart failure. *J Cardiovasc Pharmacol Therap., 11,* 31-45.

[78] Dhalla, N. S., Saini, H. K., Tappia, P. S., Sethi, R., Mengi, S. A. & Gupta, S. K. (2007). Potential role and mechanisms of subcellular remodeling in cardiac dysfunction due to ischemic heart disease. *J Cardiovasc Med., 8,* 238-50.

[79] Teerlink, J. R. (2009). A novel approach to improve cardiac performance: cardiac myosin activators. *Heart Fail Rev., 14,* 289-98.

[80] deGoma, E. M., Vagelos, R. H., Fowler, M. B. & Ashley, E. A. (2006). Emerging therapies for the management of decompensated heart failure. *J Am Coll Cardiol., 48,* 2397-409.

[81] Kahn, H., Metra, M., Blair, J. E., Vogel, M., Gheorghiade, M. et al. (2009). Istatoxime, a first in class new chemical entity exhibiting SERCA-2 activation and Na-K-ATPase inhibition: a new promising treatment for acute heart failure syndromes? *Heart Fail Rev., 14,* 277-87.

[82] Gheorghiade, M., Blair, J. E. A., Filippatos, G. S., Kremastinos, D., Valentini, G. et al.(2008). Hemodynamic, echocardiographic, and neurohormonal effects of istaroxime, a novel intravenous inotropic and lusitropic agent. *J Am Coll Cardiol., 51,* 2276-85.

[83] Kelso, E. J., McDermott, B. J. & Silke, B. (1995). Actions of the novel vasodilator, flosequinan, in isolated ventricular cardiomyocytes. *J Cardiovasc Pharmacol., 25,* 376-86.

[84] Packer, M., Narahara, K. A., Elkayam, U., Sullivan, J. M. & Creager, M. A. et al. (1993). Double-blind, placebo-controlled study of the efficacy of flosequinan in patients with chronic heart failure. Principal investigators of REFLECT study. *J Am Coll Cardiol., 22,* 65-72.

[85] Isnard, R., Lechat, P., Pousset, F., Carayon, A. & Komajda, M. et al. (1997). Hemodynamic and neurohormonal effects of flosequinan in patients with heart failure. *Fundam Clin Pharmacol., 11,* 83-9.

[86] Massie, B. M., Berk, M. R., Brozena, S. C., Elkayam, U. & Packer, M. et al. (1993). Can further benefit be achieved by adding flosequinan to patients with congestive heart failure who remain symptomatic on diuretic, digoxin, and an angiotensin converting enzyme inhibitor? Results of the flosequinan-ACE inhibitor trial (FACET). *Circulation., 88,* 492-501.

[87] Sudo, R. T., Zapata-Sudo, G. & Barreiro, E. J. (2001). The new compound, LASSBio *294,* increases the contractility of intact and

saponin-skinned cardiac muscle from wistar rats. *Br J Pharmacol., 134,* 603-13.

[88] Silva, C. L., Noel, F. & Barreiro, E. J. (2002). Cyclic GMP-dependent vasodilatory properties of LASSBio 294 in rat aorta. *Br J Pharmacol., 135,* 293-8.

In: Heart Failure: Symptoms, Causes...   ISBN: 978-1-61668-959-9
Editor: Madison S. Wright, pp. 29-49   © 2010 Nova Science Publishers, Inc.

Chapter 2

NON INVASIVE ASSESSMENT
OF MYOCARDIAL VIABILITY

Owais Khawaja,[1, 3] *Mouaz H Al-Mallah*[2, 3]*

[1] Department of Internal Medicine, Providence Hospital, Southfield, MI
[2] Henry Ford Health System, Detroit, MI
[3] Department of Internal Medicine, Wayne State University School of
Medicine,
Detroit, MI

ABSTRACT

Heart failure (HF) is a major and growing public health problem in
the United States of America (USA). Approximately 5 million patients in
USA have HF, and over 550,000 new cases are diagnosed with HF each
year. The current guidelines recommend cardiac catheterization to rule
out Coronary Artery Disease (CAD) as the cause of newly diagnosed HF
(Class I or IIa recommendation depending on the clinical scenario).
Although cardiac catheterization is the gold standard in ruling out CAD,
it does not provide information on viability and recovery of left
ventricular function post revascularization. Determining the viability of

* Corresponding author: Mouaz Al-Mallah, MD, MSc, FACC, Associate Professor of Medicine,
Wayne State University, Co-Director, Advanced Cardiovascular Imaging, Henry Ford
Hospital, 2799 West Grand Boulevard, K14, Detroit, MI 48202, Tel: 313 916 2721, Fax: 313
916 1249, Email: malmall1@hfhs.org

myocardium is therefore of great clinical significance in clinical setting. Although presence of angina in patients with severe coronary vascular disease and severe left ventricular dysfunction can signify some viable myocardium, the absence of angina does not exclude the possibility of myocardial viability in similar patient population. Echocardiography and ventriculography by itself also cannot distinguish between viable and non-viable areas of myocardium as akinetic and dyskinetic areas have been seen to completely recover following revascularization. Several advanced non-invasive modalities have been developed to rule out CAD and to determine myocardial viability in patients with heart failure. The techniques most commonly used to identify viable myocardium include Thallium-201 Single-Photon Emission Computed Tomography (^{201}Tl SPECT), Technetium-99m Sestamibi imaging (Tc-99m Sestamibi), Low Dose Dobutamine Echocardiography (LDDE), Positron Emission Tomography (PET) using a combination of flow and metabolic tracer and Cardiac Magnetic Resonance imaging (CMR). Coronary Computed Tomography Angiography (CCTA) is a non invasive tool to assess coronary anatomy. The strength of CCTA lies in its very high negative predictive value; however, it does not determine the functional significance of stenosis. CCTA use in assessment of viability is currently being evaluated in multiple research studies. Extent of myocardial Thallium-201 uptake on ^{201}Tl SPECT determines the viability of myocardial tissue and thereby helps in predicting recovery post revascularization. Flouro-I8 deoxyglucose (FDG) is a metabolic tracer used in PET for determination of viability of myocardial tissue. Normal FDG uptake in areas of decreased myocardial perfusion determines the probability of myocardial recovery in those areas post revascularization. LDDE helps to determine the myocardial viability by demonstrating stress induced contractile reserve with a high specificity. This section therefore focuses on the utilization of different imaging methods to assess the myocardial viability. It also discusses the advantages and the disadvantages of different imaging techniques. The best approach depends on the individual patient and on the expertise of the reader.

INTRODUCTION

Heart failure (HF) is a major and growing public health problem in the United States of America (USA). Approximately 5 million patients in USA have HF while over 550,000 new cases are diagnosed with HF each year [1]. The current guidelines recommend cardiac catheterization to rule out Coronary Artery Disease (CAD) as the cause of newly diagnosed HF (Class I or IIa recommendation depending on the clinical scenario). Although cardiac catheterization is the gold standard in ruling out CAD, it does not provide information on viability and recovery of left ventricular function post revascularization. Determining the viability of myocardium is of great clinical significance in clinical setting. Although presence of angina in patients with severe coronary vascular disease and severe left ventricular dysfunction can signify some viable myocardium [2], the absence of angina does not exclude the possibility of myocardial viability in similar patient population. Echocardiography and ventriculography by itself also cannot distinguish between viable and non-viable areas of myocardium as akinetic and dyskinetic areas have been seen to completely recover following revascularization. Several advanced non-invasive modalities have been developed to rule out CAD and to determine myocardial viability in patients with heart failure. There are varieties of clinical markers that can be assessed for the determination of myocardial viability with each having its own strength and weaknesses as shown in table 1. The techniques most commonly used to identify viable myocardium include Thallium-201 Single-Photon Emission Computed Tomography (^{201}Tl SPECT), Technetium-99m Sestamibi imaging (Tc-99m Sestamibi), Low Dose Dobutamine Echocardiography (LDDE), Positron Emission Tomography (PET) and Cardiac Magnetic Resonance imaging (CMR). Coronary Computed Tomography Angiography (CCTA) is a non invasive tool to assess coronary anatomy.

Table 1. Clinical Markers of Viability and Imaging Modalities

	EKG	ECHO	^{201}SPECT	PET	CMR
Q waves	+				
Metabolic Function				+	
Myocyte Integrity			+	+	+
Altered Tissue Composition					+
Perfusion			+	+	+
No or low reflow					+
Wall Thickness		+	+/-	+/-	+
Wall motion		+	+/-	+/-	++

Abbreviations: EKG: Electrocardiogram; ECHO: Echocardiography; ^{201}Tl SPECT: Thallium-201 Single Photon emission Computed Tomography PET: Positron Emission Tomography; CMR: Cardiac Magnetic Resonance

Its strength of this technique lies in its very high negative predictive value; however, it does not determine the functional significance of stenosis. CCTA use in assessment of viability is currently being evaluated in multiple research studies. This chapter therefore focuses on the utilization of imaging methods to assess the myocardial viability. It also discusses the advantages and the disadvantages of different imaging techniques.

PATHOPHYSIOLOGICAL MECHANISMS OF VIABILITY

Identification of viability in myocardial tissue is of great clinical significance. Patients with triple vessel coronary artery disease and depressed Left Ventricular Ejection Fraction (LVEF) have been shown to have improved survival with Coronary Artery Bypass Grafting (CABG) [3, 4].

The term *hibernating myocardium* was thereby used to describe such chronic Left Ventricular (LV) dysfunction that improved partially or completely following revascularization and/or decrease in the myocardial oxygen demand [5, 6]. The concept behind this improvement was that with chronic ischemia the tissue metabolism decreases thereby decreasing the tissue energy demands and thus limiting irreversible tissue damage. This concept however has been questioned by recent studies demonstrating normal perfusion and metabolism in hibernating myocardial segments [7-10].

Subsequently the concept of *myocardial stunning* was introduced to describe reversible prolonged mechanical dysfunction following brief period of reduced coronary blood flow even after reestablishment of coronary flow and lack of tissue damage [11]. The functional recovery in humans may take days to weeks [12]. Potential explanations proposed for myocardial stunning including the generation of reactive oxygen radicals secondary to tissue ischemia with resultant oxidant stress or disturbed cellular calcium homeostasis with reduction in myocardial contractility [13-16].

One other proposed theory for hibernating myocardial region has been repetitive episodes of myocardial stunning [7, 11, 17]. Whether myocardial stunning and hibernation are two separate entities or represent same entity for now remains unclear [12]. Multiple modalities that can be used to assess myocardial viability are reviewed below.

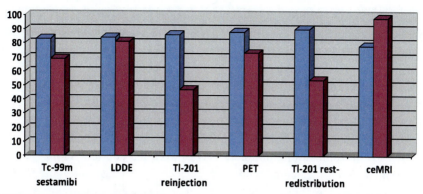

* Blue Bar represents sensitivity
* Purple Bar represents specificity
Abbreviations: Tc-99m sestamibi: Technitium-99m sestamibi; LDDE: Low Dose
    Dobutamine Echocardiography; Tl-201: Thallium-201; PET: Positron Emission
    Tomography; ceMRI: contrast enhanced Magnetic Resonance Imaging
Figure Legend. Bar chart comparing the sensitivities and specificities of various non
    invasive imaging modalities in the assessment of myocardial viability.

Figure 1. Relative Accuracy of Viability Detection with different Imaging Modalities

THALLIUM-201 SINGLE-PHOTON EMISSION COMPUTED TOMOGRAPHY (^{201}TL SPECT)

Thallium-201 is radioactive potassium analog with a prolonged half-life
(~73 hours). It has a high myocardial extraction rate with rate remaining
constant under basal conditions as well as following increased heart rate [18].
Its uptake by myocardium indicates viable myocardium. Following initial
extraction by myocardial cells Thallium-201 than begins to leak out of the
myocardial cells into the coronary circulation depending on the rate of
coronary blood flow called "differential washout". This allows for assessment
of coronary blood flow during rest and post stress states [19]. Redistribution of
Thallium-201 in areas that initially had a defect in Thallium-201 uptake is
critically important in determining the viability of myocardial tissue with this
technique. Traditionally ^{201}Tl SPECT with rest and 3-4 hours delayed images
have been used for the determination of myocardial viability. Newer
techniques have been developed for enhancing the detection of viable
myocardium including reinjection of Thallium-201 and 24 hour delayed
imaging.

Reinjection of Thallium-201following the delayed redistribution image is essential since defect reversibility as seen with this technique is dependent on plasma concentration of the isotope. Therefore increasing the plasma concentration of isotope by reinjection might increase the uptake in previously ischemic areas. Enhanced Thallium-201 uptake has been demonstrated in 30-50% of segments following the reinjection that were initially noted as fixed defects on 4 hour delayed imaging with single injection study [20-22].

Delayed imaging technique is needed since more than 3-4 hours are required for the isotope to equilibrate between plasma and the viable areas of myocardium. Such a phenomenon of delayed redistribution at 24 hours has been demonstrated in about 20-60% of fixed defects seen with 4 hour imaging with improved uptake following the coronary revascularization [23, 24].

^{201}Tl SPECT has been found to be very helpful in detecting the presence of viable myocardium, however it does not always translates into recovery with improved wall motion abnormality post revascularization [25]. Reasons for this limitation are various including but not limited to the detection of injured myocardial cells of not sufficient size to improve wall motion abnormality, scar tissue limiting the wall motion of adjacent viable myocardium, viable myocardium in subepicardial layer with necrotic tissue in subendocardium and inadequate functional recovery in 3 months [26, 27].

Sensitivity and specificity of different nuclear and non-nuclear imaging modalities for assessing the myocardial viability is shown in figure 1. In conclusion ^{201}Tl SPECT has a high sensitivity but low specificity in predicting the recovery of myocardial functional capacity post revascularization.

TECHNETIUM-99M SESTAMIBI IMAGING (TC-99M SESTAMIBI/ CARDIOLITE^{TM})

Tc-99m is a generator produced product with a half life of six hours and is easily available on site in most of the places. Tc-99m sestamibi belongs to the isonitrile group of compounds. It is transferred passively across the plasma and mitochondrial membranes with predominant sequestration in the mitochondria [28]. The first pass myocardial extraction for Tc-99m sestamibi has been shown to be less than that of Thallium-201 [29]. Tc-99m sestamibi myocardial uptake has been shown to be proportional to blood flow within normal limits (Figure 2). It undergoes minimal redistribution over time [30, 31]. Tracer uptake in areas with reduced coronary flow and partial myocardial damage is affected more so by flow than by injury itself as has been shown in studies with apparently necrotic area on Tc-99m rest scan gaining functional recovery following revascularization [32]. Tc-99m thereby can underestimate the viability as shown in several human studies as compared to other nuclear imaging methods [33-35]. A possible way to counter act this phenomenon would be to administer vasodilator agent like Nitrate along with Tc-99m sestamibi which can improve the coronary blood flow [36-42]. This thereby can enhance Tc-99m sestamibi tracer uptake by the hypoperfused though viable myocardial tissue [43]. In spite of the lack of redistribution Tc-99m sestamibi can still be used to detect viable myocardium and predict post revascularization functional improvement, this again can be further enhanced by Nitrate administration prior to the tracer injection [44-47].

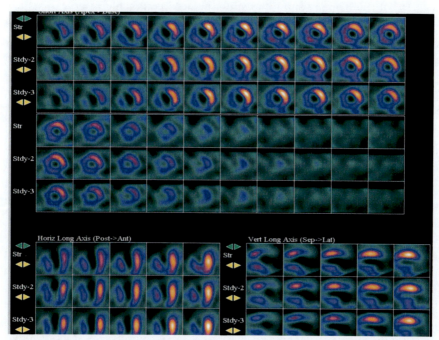

Figure Legend: The top raw indicates stress images, the middle raw (study -2) indicates rest perfusion and the lower raw (study -3) indicates late images. In this patient, there is evidence of a large inferior, septal and inferolateral fixed perfusion defect with no evidence of ischemia or viability.

Figure 2. Tc-99m Sestamibi Stress Rest Viability Scan

Following irreversible injury to myocardium the membrane potentials are altered and that in turn inhibits the cellular uptake and retention of Tc-99m sestamibi. Tc-99m sestamibi also has better physical characteristics for gamma camera producing better images as compared to Thallium-201 [48].

LOW-DOSE DOBUTAMINE ECHOCARDIOGRAPHY (LDDE)

The wide availability and portability of echocardiography makes it a popular testing modality. Dobutamine is a sympathomimetic agent acting predominantly on β_1 receptors and is used in the treatment of patients with congestive heart failure and cardiogenic shock. Viability can be determined with LDDE by demonstrating the stress induced contractile reserve. This can be done using incremental doses of dobutamine with improved contractility in the viable myocardial tissue at low doses while regression in the contractility at higher doses [49]. Recently high dose dobutamine infusion protocol with infusion of atropine if needed have been developed. Following the high dose dobutamine infusion protocol four possible myocardial contractile patterns can be seen i.e. initial improvement and then worsening of myocardial contractility; worsening of myocardial contractility without any initial improvement; sustained improvement in myocardial contractility and no change in the myocardial contractility. First pattern represents myocardial ischemia with viable myocardial tissue, second pattern represents severe myocardial ischemia, third pattern represents subendocardial necrosis while the fourth response pattern represents transmural scar of the myocardium. Dobutamine has also been shown to be helpful in differentiating irreversibly injured areas from stunned/hibernating areas of myocardium demonstrating improved contractility following dobutamine infusion [50]. Patients with significant increase in cardiac contractility following dobutamine infusion i.e. increase in LVEF >10%, have been shown to have improved LV function and long term survival following coronary revascularization [51]. Addition of Tissue Doppler Imaging (TDI) has also been shown to improve the sensitivity of LDDE in the detection of hibernating myocardium [52]. Improved wall thickness pattern in dyssynergic segments following infusion of low dose dobutamine has also been shown to be a good predictor for improved wall motion abnormality following revascularization [25]. Dobutamine echocardiography has been shown to have a concordance rate of 68% with ^{201}Tl SPECT. Panza et al in their study demonstrated 30% of myocardial tissue to be non-viable on LDDE that was deemed to be viable on ^{201}Tl SPECT, while in 2% of cases LDDE demonstrated viability in terms of contractile reserve for the myocardial tissue that was deemed non-viable on ^{201}Tl SPECT [53]. Thus the particular benefit of LDDE in comparison to nuclear methods of assessing viability is in its ability to detect viability in terms of contractile reserve. However, it is limited by qualitative assessment and high inter-observer variability.

POSITRON EMISSION TOMOGRAPHY (PET)

PET is an advanced imaging modality introduced and has been claimed to be the gold standard technique for the determination of myocardial viability. The basic principle of this technique involves radioactive tracer rubidium-82 or nitrogen-13 ammonia used as perfusion tracers and flouro-18 deoxyglucose (FDG) used as a metabolic tracer. During the fasting state plasma Free Fatty Acids (FFA) constitute the major energy producing fuel for the myocardial tissue [54]. However during the fed state with increase in the plasma glucose and insulin levels there is increased cellular transport of glucose into the cells, with glucose than serving as major energy producing fuel for the myocardial tissue [55]. FFA metabolism is highly sensitive to the availability of oxygen which when declines in conditions like myocardial ischemia; metabolism of glucose markedly increases by ischemic myocardial tissue [56-58]. This thereby helps in the differentiation of viable from the non viable myocardial tissue that is identified by reduced perfusion along with decreased FDG uptake, while the regions with viable myocardial tissue demonstrate normal FDG uptake with low perfusion (Figure 3). Patterns of left ventricular function (global and regional) as obtained from the gated PET images correspond with that of CMR [59]. Increased left ventricular volume and cavity size correspond with poor outcome with respect to left ventricular function and survival even with evidence of myocardial viability [60]. PET identified viability was demonstrated to be associated with improved post revascularization prognosis; however this was same as that noted with LDDE [61], ^{201}Tl SPECT [62] and CMR [63].

Di Carli et al studied the myocardial viability with PET in patients with severely depressed LVEF. In a study of 36 patients with LVEF 28 +/- 6 , the greatest benefit in heart failure symptom following revascularization was seen in the patients with large perfusion-metabolism **mismatches (defined as ≥** 18%) [64].

Beanlands et al [65] **in their** 'Positron emission tomography and recovery following revascularization' (PARR-1) study demonstrated the importance of scar tissue identification on PET and its correlation with predicted improvement in the LVEF. Myocardial scar tissue as seen on PET scan was quantified as small (0% - 16%), moderate (16% - 27.5%) and large (27.5% - 47%). Following the revascularization at three months LVEF improved by 9.0% ± 1.9% for patients with small amount of scar tissue, 3.7% ± 1.6% for patients with moderate amount of scar tissue and only 1.3% ± 1.5% for patients with large amount of scar tissue. On comparing the improvement in LVEF in patients with small versus large amount of myocardial scarring the 'p' value was significant at 0.003. Quantification of the scar tissue in this study was found to be an independent predictor of improvement in the LVEF even after adjusting for all the confounding variables.

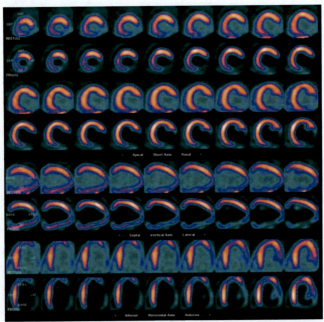

Figure Legend. The top raw indicates perfusion images, and the lower raw (study -3) indicates viability FDG images. In this patient, there is evidence of a large inferior, and inferolateral matched perfusion defect with no evidence of viability.

Figure 3. PET Viability Assessment Study

Recently, Beanlands et al [66] in their 'F-18-Fluorodeoxyglucose Positron Emission Tomography Imaging-Assisted Management of Patients With Severe Left Ventricular Dysfunction and Suspected Coronary Disease' (PARR-2) study evaluated whether PET evaluation of the viability of myocardial tissue can be used to guide the revascularization decision. The study failed to show any significant advantage of using PET assisted management decision versus standard decision making process with respect to the incidence of myocardial infarction, recurrent admissions secondary to cardiac causes or cardiovascular death at one year. However, this was because nearly one third of the patients enrolled in the study did not follow the PET recommended therapy. When adherent patients were analyzed, it was evident that PET guided therapy can be used to guide the revascularization decisions.

An important limitation with FDG use is that the image quality for patients with impaired glucose tolerance or overt diabetes could be poor. The widespread use of PET is also limited by its operative cost, availability of tracers used along with unfamiliarity with the interpretation of image.

CARDIAC MAGNETIC RESONANCE IMAGING (CMR)

CMR is also a new and evolving imaging modality that involves real time images of myocardial contractility with enhanced image quality (Figure 4). It provides reproducible and accurate estimation of ventricular sizes, volume, wall thickness and mass apart from the estimation of LVEF [67]. Another advantage of CMR is that it can be applied in three dimensions so the assessment of wall motion can be done in circumferential as well as radial and longitudinal directions [68, 69]. Contrast enhanced MRI (ceMRI) with gadolinium-DTPA was first described in 1984 and is very useful in detecting the areas of infarction which appear to be hyper enhanced on ceMRI (Figure 5). These hyper enhanced areas have been shown to correlate well with fixed thallium defect size on ^{201}Tl SPECT as shown in a study conducted by Lima, et al [70]. Kim et al [71] evaluated the patterns of myocardial damage following coronary occlusion as seen on ceMRI. Their study demonstrated hyper enhancement in infracted areas of myocardium (acute or chronic) while no such phenomenon was seen in the reversibly damaged area of myocardium. Kim et al [63] in another study evaluated the role of detection of myocardial scar tissue with ceMRI and the prediction of improvement in LVEF following revascularization. They found strong correlation between decrease in the improvement of myocardial contractility post revascularization and increase in the extent of transmural hyper enhancement on ceMRI pre operatively. Contractility increased post revascularization in 78% of segments with no hyper enhancement versus in only 1.7% of segments with hyper enhancement on ceMRI prior to the revascularization procedure. Various other studies have also demonstrated no increase in the gadolinium concentration or enhancement with ceMRI in the areas of reversibly injured myocardial tissue suggesting that the enhanced areas visible on ceMRI represent non viable irreversibly injured myocardium [72, 73]. Contrast enhancement, however, is not specific for ischemia; it can also be seen with inflammatory and infiltrative diseases though the pattern of enhancement is different from that seen with ischemia or infarction. The use of CMR has been limited by various factors including lack of availability and expertise at various centers, presence of cardiac defibrillators and other metallic devices in human body. It cannot be used in patients with advanced renal failure owing to the possibility of developing a serious condition called Nephrogenic Systemic Fibrosis following exposure to gadolinium used for the contrast enhancement.

CARDIAC COMPUTED TOMOGRAPHY ANGIOGRAPHY (CCTA)

CCTA has increasingly been used for non invasive assessment of coronary vasculature. Few studies have also looked into its application for assessment of myocardial viability however it is not the main utility of CCTA at this point of time. Left ventricular end diastolic wall thickness can be used as a viability criteria. Studies have evaluated the concordance of contrast enhanced CCTA and ceMRI for the detection of viability of myocardial tissue. In general, there is underestimation of infarct size with the contrast enhanced CCTA as compared to that with ceMRI [74]. Another study by Mahnken et al. however demonstrated good concordance between the contrast enhanced CCTA and ceMRI [75].

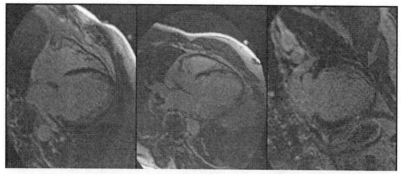

Figure Legend. MRI delayed enhancement imaging in 4 chambers, 3 chambers and 2 chambers imaging. There is evidence of a small area of subendocardial delayed enhancement <50% of wall thickness in the anterior wall. This indicates viability and tendency toward functional recovery with revascularization. Red Arrow pointing towards area of endocardial scarring.

Figure 4. Predominantly Viable Myocardium as seen on CMR

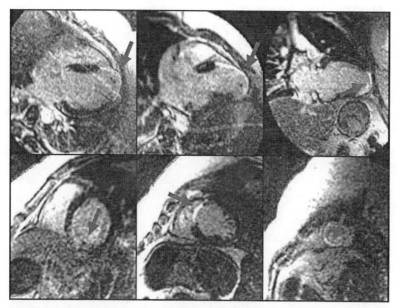

Figure Legend. MRI delayed enhancement imaging in 4 chambers, 3 chambers and 2 chambers as well as short axis. There is evidence of a large area of transmural delayed enhancement >50% of wall thickness in the LAD territory wall. This indicates lack of viability Red Arrow pointing towards area of scarring.

Figure 5. Hyper enhancement as seen on ceMRI

The growth in the number of PET cameras worldwide, offers new opportunities for the integration of PET and 64 Slice Computed Tomography (CT) technology. Such a study would in one test determine the etiology of HF, define the extent of reversible and irreversible ventricular dysfunction based on the metabolic evaluation of the left ventricular myocardium [76]. However, an important limitation with this modality however remains the use of contrast agent in patients with impaired renal function, which frequently is the case in patients with advanced heart failure as well as the issues linked to excessive radiation exposure. The usefulness of CCTA for the determination of myocardial viability remains controversial for now until further prospective studies are conducted.

CONCLUSION

The assessment of myocardial viability is an integral part of the diagnostic and prognostic work up of patients with congestive heart failure predominantly secondary to impaired coronary perfusion. One important limitation is that most of these viability studies (>90%) available were done on patients with LVEF of $\geq$ 30% with good predictable outcomes based on the imaging studies [77]. This however might not be the case in patients with highest clinical risk i.e. LVEF $\leq$ 30%, where the accuracy of the viability testing including that done with PET significantly declines [78]. Different non invasive imaging modalities have their own advantages and disadvantages in specific patient populations as discussed above. The best approach therefore depends on the individual patient itself and on the expertise of the reader.

REFERENCES

[1]   American Heart Association. Heart disease and stroke statistics - 2007 update. Dallas, Texas: *American Heart Association*, 2007.

[2]   Romero-Farina, G; C R. J; Aguadé-Bruix, S, et al, Influence of chronic angina prior to infarction in the diagnosis of viability and left ventricular remodelling in myocardial perfusion gated-SPECT. *Rev Esp Med Nucl.*, 2008, 27(4), 245-252.

[3]   Chatterjee, K; SH; Parmley, WW; et al, Influence of direct myocardial revascularization on left ventricular asynergy and function in patients

with coronary heart disease: with and without previous myocardial infarction. *Circulation*, 1973, 47, 276-286.

[4] Rees, G; BJ; Kremkau, EL; et al, Influence of aortocoronary bypass surgery on left ventricular performance. *N Engl J Med*; 1971, 284, 1116-1120.

[5] Diamond, GA; FJ; deLuz, PL; et al, Post-extrasystolic potentiation of ischemic myocardium by atrial stimulation. *Am Heart J*, 1978, 95, 204-209.

[6] SH, R., The hibernating myocardium. *Am Heart J*, 1989, 117, 211-221.

[7] Vanoverschelde, JL; WW; Depre, C; et al, Mechanisms of chronic regional postischemic dysfunction in humans: new insights from the study of noninfarcted collateral-dependent myocardium. *Circulation*, 1993, 87, 1513-1523.

[8] Marinho, NV; KB; Costa, DC; et al, Pathophysiology of chronic left ventricular dysfunction: new insights from the measurement of absolute myocardial blood flow and glucose utilization. *Circulation*, 1996, 737-744.

[9] Conversano, A; WJ; Geltman, EM; et al, Delineation of myocardial stunning and hibernation by positron emission tomography in advanced coronary artery disease. *Am Heart J*, 1996, 131, 440-450.

[10] Gerber, BL; VJ; Bol, A, et al, Myocardial blood flow, glucose uptake, and recruitment of inotropic reserve in chronic left ventricular ischemic dysfunction: implications for the pathophysiology of chronic myocardial hibernation. *Circulation*, 1996, 94, 651-659.

[11] Braunwald, E; KR. The stunned myocardium: prolonged, postischemic ventricular dysfunction. *Circulation*, 1982, 66, 1146-1149.

[12] Kloner, RA; BR; Marbán, E, et al, Medical and cellular implications of stunning, hibernation, and preconditioning: an NHLBI workshop. *Circulation*, 1998, 97, 1848-1867.

[13] R, B. Mechanism of myocardial "stunning". *Circulation*, 1990, 82(723-738).

[14] Bolli, R; ME. Molecular and cellular mechanisms of myocardial stunning. *Physiol Rev.*, 1999, 79, 609-634.

[15] Kusuoka, H; ME. Cellular mechanisms of myocardial stunning. *Annu Rev Physiol.*, 1992, 54, 243-256.

[16] Marbán, E; KY. Corretti M, et al, Calcium and its role in myocardial cell injury during ischemia and reperfusion. *Circulation*, 1989, 80, IV17-IV22.

[17] Shen, YT; VS. Mechanism of impaired myocardial function during progressive coronary stenosis in conscious pigs: hibernation versus stunning? *Circ Res.*, 1995, 76, 479-488.

[18] Weich, HF; SH; Pitt, B. The extraction of thallium-201 by the myocardium. *Circulation*, 1977, 56(2), 188-191.

[19] Pohost, GM; ZL;. Moore, RH; et al, Differentiation of transiently ischemic from infarcted myocardium by serial imaging after a single dose of thallium-201. *Circulation*, 1977, 55(2), 294-302.

[20] Dilsizian, V; RT; Freedman, NMT. et al, Enhanced detection of ischemic but viable myocardium by the reinjection of thallium after stress-redistribution imaging. *N Engl J Med.*, 1990, 323, 141-146.

[21] Rocco, Tp; DV; McKusick, KA; et al, Comparison of thallium redistribution with rest "reinjection" imaging for the detection of viable myocardium. *Am J Cardiol*, 1990, 66, 158-163.

[22] Ohtani, H; TN; Yonekura, Y; et al, Value of thallium-201 reinjection after delayed SPECT imaging for predicting reversible ischemia after coronary artery bypass grafting. *Am J Cardiol*, 1990, 66, 394-399.

[23] Kiat, H; BD; Maddahi, J; et al, Late reversibility of tomographic myocardial thallium-201 defects: An accurate marker of myocardial viability. *JAm Coll Cardiol*, 1988, 12, 1456-1463.

[24] Yang, LD; BD; Kiat, H; et al, The frequency of late reversibility in SPECT thallium-201 stress-redistributions tudies. *J Am Coll Cardiol*, 1990, 15, 334-340.

[25] Arnese, M; CJ; Salustri, A; Maat, APWM; et al, Prediction of Improvement of Regional Left Ventricular Function After Surgical Revascularization Circulation, 1995, 91, 2748-2752.

[26] Bashour, TT; M.D. Myocardial hibernation and `embalment. *Am Heart J*, 1990, 119, 706-708.

[27] Sklenar, J; IS; Villanueva, FS; et al, Dobutamine echocardiography for determining the extent of myocardial salvage after reperfusion, an experimental evaluation. *Circulation*, 1994, 90, 1502-1512.

[28] ML; PWDKJC. Uptake and retention of hexakis (2-methoxyisobutyl isonitrile) technetium(I) in cultured chick myocardial cells. Mitochondrial and plasma membrane potential dependence. *Circulation*, 1990, 82(5), 1826-1838.

[29] DJ; LJM. Comparison of the myocardial uptake of a technetium-labeled isonitrile analogue and thallium. *Circ Res.*, 1989, 65(3), 632-639.

[30] Okada, RD; GD; Gaffney, T; et al, Myocardial kinetics of technetium-99m-hexakis-2-methoxy-2-methylpropyl-isonitrile. *Circulation*, 1988, 77(2), 491-498.

[31] Glover, DK; OR. Myocardial kinetics of Tc-MIBI in canine myocardium after dipyridamole. *Circulation*, 1990, 81(2), 628-637.

[32] Marzullo, P; SG; Parodi, 0. The role ofsestamibi scintigraphy in the radioisotopic assessment of myocardial viability. *J Nucl Med*, 1992, 33, 1925-1930.

[33] Dilsizian, V; Arrighi, IA; D; et al, Myocardial viability in patients with chronic coronary artery disease. Comparison of @â€œTc-sestamibi with thallium reinjection and [18F fluorodeoxyglucose. *Circulation*, 1994, 89, 578-587.

[34] Cuocolo, A; PL. Ricciardelli B, et al, Identification of viable myocardium in patients with chronic coronary artery disease: comparison of thallium-201 scintigraphy with reinjection and technetium-99m-methoxyisobutyl isonitrile. *J Nucl Cardiol*, 1992, 33, 505-511.

[35] Altenhoefer, C; KHi; DOrr, R. et al, Fluorine-18 deoxyglucose PET for the assessment of viable myocardium in perfusion defects in 99mTc-MIBI SPECT: a comparative study in patients with coronary artery disease. *Eur J Nucl Med*, 1992, 19, 334-342.

[36] Cohn, PF; MD; Holman, BL; et al, Effect of sublingually administered nitroglycerin on regional myocardial blood flow in patients with coronary artery disease. *Am J Cardiol*, 1977, 39, 672-678.

[37] Cohen, MV; SE; Kirk, ES. Comparative effects of nitroglycerin and isosorbide dinitrate on coronary collateral vessels and ischemic myocardium in dogs. *Am J Cardiol*, 1976, 37, 244-249.

[38] Brown, BG; BEPR., et al, The mechanism of nitroglycerin action: stenosis vasodilation as a major component of the drug response. *Circulation*, 1981, 64, 1089-1097.

[39] Feldman, RI; CC. Relief of myocardial ischemia with nitroglycerin: what is the mechanism? . *Circulation*, 1981, 64, 1098-1100.

[40] BG; B. Response of normal and diseased epicardial coronary arteries to vasoactive drugs: quantitative arteriographic studies. *Am J Cardiol*, 1985, 56, 23E-29E.

[41] Fujita, M; YK; Hirai, T; et al Significance ofcollateral circulation in reversible left ventricular asynergy by nitroglycerin in patients with relatively recent myocardial infarction. *Am Heart J*, 1990, 120, 521-528.

[42] Aoki, M; SK; Koyanagi, S; et al, Effect of nitroglycerin on coronary collateral function during exercise evaluated by quantitative analysis of thallium-201 SPECT. *Am Heart J*, 1991, 121(1361).

[43] Bisi, G; SR; Santoro, GM; et al, Sublingual isosorbide dinitrate to improve 99mTc..teboroxime perfusion defect reversibility. *J Nucl Med.*, 1994, 35, 1274-1278.

[44] Udelson, JE; CP; Metherall, J; et al Predicting recovery of severe regional ventricular dysfunction. Comparison of resting scintigraphy with 201Tl and 99mTc-sestamibi. *Circulation*, 1994, 89(6), 2552-2561.

[45] Maurea, S; CA; Soricelli, A; et al, Enhanced detection of viable myocardium by technetium-99m-MIBI imaging after nitrate administration in chronic coronary artery disease. *J Nucl Med*, 1995, 36(11), 1945-1952.

[46] Bisi, G; SR; Santoro, GM; et al, Technetium-99m-sestamibi imaging with nitrate infusion to detect viable hibernating myocardium and predict postrevascularization recovery. *J Nucl Med*, 1995, 36(11), 1994-2000.

[47] Sciagra, R; BG; Santoro, GM; et al, Comparison of baseline-nitrate technetium-99m sestamibi with rest-redistribution thallium-201 tomography in detecting viable hibernating myocardium and predicting postrevascularization recovery. *J Am Coll Cardiol*, 1997, 30(2), 384-391.

[48] Beller, GA; WD. Physiologic basis of myocardial perfusion imaging with the technetium-99m agents. *Semin Nucl Med*, 1991, 21, 173-181.

[49] Picano, E; BdSM; de Moura Duarte, LF; et al, Detection of viable myocardium by dobutamine and dipyridamole stress echocardiography. *Herz*, 1994, 19, 204-209.

[50] Pemne-Filardi, P; BS; Dilsizian, V, et al, Metabolic evidence of viable myocardium in regions with reduced wall thickness and absent wall thickening in patients with chronic ischemic left ventricular dysfunction. *J Am Coll Cardiol*, 1992, 20, 161-168.

[51] Nesto, RW; CL; Collins, JJ; et al, Inotropic contractile reserve: a useful predictor of increased 5-year survival and improved postoperative left ventricular function in patients with coronary artery disease and reduced ejection fraction. *Am J Cardiol*, 1982, 50, 39-44.

[52] Hoffmann, R; AE; Nowak, B; et al, Strain rate measurement by Doppler echocardiography allows improved assessment of myocardial viability inpatients with depressed left ventricular function. *J Am Coll Cardiol*, 2002, 39, 443-449.

[53] Panza, JA; DV; Laurienzo, JM; et al, Relation Between Thallium Uptake and Contractile Response to Dobutamine Circulation, 1995, 91, 990-998.

[54] LH, O. The Heart. *Physiology and Metabolism*. Second ed. New York: Raven Press, 1991.

[55] Young, LH; CD; Russell, RR; et al, Cellular and molecular regulation of cardiac glucose transport. *J Nucl Cardiol*, 2000, 7, 267-276.

[56] LH, O. Effects of regional ischemia on metabolism of glucose and fatty acids. *Circ Res.*, 1976, 38, 152-174.

[57] AJ, L. Alterations of carbohydrate and lipid metabolism in the acutely ischemic heart. *Progr Cardiovasc Dis.*, 1981, 23, 321-326.

[58] Camici, P; AL; Spinks, T; et al Increase uptake of 18F-fluorodeoxyglucose in postischemic myocardium of patients with exercise-induced angina. *Circulation*, 1986, 74, 81-88.

[59] Schaefer, WM; LC; Nowak, B; et al, Validation of an evaluation routine for left ventricular volumes, ejection fraction and wall motion from gated cardiac FDG PET: a comparison with cardiac magnetic resonance imaging. *Eur J Nucl Med Mol Imaging*, 2003, 30, 545-553.

[60] Yamaguchi, A; I; T; Adachi, H; et al, Left ventricular volume predicts postoperative course in patients with ischemic cardiomyopathy. *Ann Thorac Surg*, 1998, 65, 434-438.

[61] Perrone-Filardi, P; PL; Prastaro, M; et al, Dobutamine echocardiography predicts improvement of hypoperfused dysfunctional myocardium after revascularization in patients with coronary artery disease. *Circulation*, 1995, 91, 2556-2565.

[62] Ragosta, M; BG; Watson, DD; et al, Quantitative planar rest-redistribution 201Tl imaging in detection of myocardial viability and prediction of improvement in left ventricular function after coronary bypass surgery in patients with severely depressed left ventricular function. *Circulation*, 1993, 87, 1630-1641.

[63] Kim, RJ; WE., Rafael, A; et al, The use of contrast-enhanced magnetic resonance imaging to identify reversible myocardial dysfunction. *N Engl J Med*, 2000, 343, 1445-1453.

[64] Di Carli, MF; AF; Schelbert, HR; et al, Quantitative Relation Between Myocardial Viability and Improvement in Heart Failure Symptoms After Revascularization in Patients With Ischemic Cardiomyopathy Circulation, 1995, 92, 3436-3444.

[65] Beanlands, B; RS; RT; deKemp, RA; et al, Positron emission tomography and recovery following revascularization (PARR-1), the importance of scar and the development of a prediction rule for the

degree of recovery of left ventricular function Am Coll Cardiol, 2002, 40, 1735-1743.

[66] Beanlands, B; NG; RS; Huszti, E; et al, F-18-Fluorodeoxyglucose Positron Emission Tomography Imaging-Assisted Management of Patients With Severe Left Ventricular Dysfunction and Suspected Coronary Disease. *J Am Coll Cardiol*, 2007, 50, 2002-2012.

[67] Chuang, ML; BR; Riley, MF; et al, Three-dimensional echocardiographic measurement of left ventricular mass: comparison with magnetic resonance imaging and two-dimensional echocardiographic determinations in man. *International journal of cardiac imaging*, 2000, 16(5), 347-357.

[68] Moore, CC; ODW; McVeigh, ER; et al, Calculation of three-dimensional left ventricular strains from biplanar tagged MR images. *J Magn Reson Imaging*, 1992, 2, 165-175.

[69] O'Dell, WG; MC; Hunter, WC; et al, Three-dimensional myocardial deformations: calculation with displacement field fitting to tagged MR images. *Radiology*, 1995, 195, 829-835.

[70] Lima, JA; JR; Bazille, A; et al, Regional heterogeneity of human myocardial infarcts demonstrated by contrast-enhanced MRI: potential mechanisms. *Circulation*, 1995, 92, 1117-1125.

[71] Kim, RJ; FD; Parrish, TB; et al, Relationship of MRI delayed contrast enhancement to irreversible injury, infarct age, and contractile function. *Circulation*, 1999, 100, 1992-2002.

[72] Rehwald, WG; FD; Chen, EL; et al, Myocardial magnetic resonance imaging contrast agent concentrations after reversible and irreversible ischemic injury. *Circulation*, 2002, 105, 224-229.

[73] McNamara, MT; TD; Revel, D; et al, Differentiation of reversible and irreversible myocardial injury by MR imaging with and without gadolinium-DTPA. *Radiology*, 1986, 158, 765-769.

[74] Nikolaou, K; SJ; Poon, M; et al, Assessment of myocardial perfusion and viability from routine contrast-enhanced 16-detector-row computed tomography of the heart: preliminary results. *Eur Radiol*, 2005, 15, 864-871.

[75] Mahnken, AH; KR; Katoh, M; et al, Assessment of myocardial viability in reperfused acute myocardial infarction using 16-slice computed tomography in comparison to magnetic resonance imaging. *J Am Coll Cardiol*, 2005, 45, 2042-2047.

[76] Schwaiger, M; ZM. Nekolla S PET/CT: Challenge for Nuclear Cardiology. *J Nucl Cardiol*, 2005, 46(10), 1664-1678.

[77] Bax, JJ; PD; Elhendy, A; et al, Sensitivity, specificity, and predictive accuracies of various noninvasive techniques for detecting hibernating myocardium. *Curr Probl Cardiol*, 2001, 26, 141-186.
[78] Di Carli, MF; DS; Meserve, J; et al, Clinical Myocardial Perfusion PET/CT. *J Nucl Med.*, 2007, 48(5), 783-793.

In: Heart Failure: Symptoms, Causes...   ISBN: 978-1-61668-959-9
Editor: Madison S. Wright, pp. 51-72   © 2010 Nova Science Publishers, Inc.

Chapter 3

HETEROTRIMERIC G PROTEINS IN HEART FAILURE

*Motohiro Nishida, Mina Ohba, Michio Nakaya and Hitoshi Kurose**

Department of Pharmacology and Toxicology, Graduate School of
Pharmaceutical Sciences, Kyushu University, 3-1-1 Maidashi, Higashi-ku,
Fukuoka 812-8582, Japan

ABSTRACT

Structural remodeling of the heart, including myocardial hypertrophy
and fibrosis, is a key determinant for the clinical outcome of heart failure.
A variety of evidence indicates the importance of neurohumoral factors,
such as endothelin-1, angiotensin II, and norepinephrine for the initial
phase of the development of cardiac remodeling. These agonists stimulate
seven transmembrane spanning receptors that are coupled to
heterotrimeric GTP-binding proteins (G proteins) of the G_i, G_q and G_{12}
subfamilies. The pathophysiological roles of each G protein-mediated
signaling have been revealed by studies using transgenic and knockout
mice. Using specific pharmacological tools to assess the involvement of
G protein signaling pathways, we have found that diacylglycerol-
activated transient receptor potential canonical (TRPC) channels (TRPC3
and TRPC6), one of the downstream effectors regulated by $G\alpha_q$, work as

---

* Corresponding author: E-mail: kurose@phar.kyushu-u.ac.jp. Tel & Fax: +81-92-642-6884

a key mediator in the development of cardiac hypertrophy. In contrast, we also revealed that activation of $G\alpha_{12}$ family proteins in cardiomyocytes mediates pressure overload-induced cardiac fibrosis. Stimulation of purinergic $P2Y_6$ receptors by extracellular nucleotides released by mechanical stretch is a trigger of $G\alpha_{12}$-mediated fibrotic responses of the heart. Although cardiac fibrosis is believed to accompany with $G\alpha_q$-mediated pathological hypertrophy that eventually results in heart failure, our results clearly show that cardiac fibrosis and hypertrophy are independent processes. These findings will provide a new insight into the molecular mechanisms underlying pathogenesis of heart failure.

INTRODUCTION

G protein-coupled receptors (GPCRs) are a conserved family of seven transmembrane spanning receptors that occupy the majority of receptors in the genome. About 50-60% of drugs which are widely used for therapeutic treatment all over the world may directly or indirectly target GPCRs [1]. Heart failure is a final stage of every cardiovascular disease. The number of patients with heart failure is estimated more than 1 million people in Japan and about 5 million people in USA, and the number has a tendency to increase year by year with aging [2]. Although it has been estimated that approximately 200 kinds of GPCRs are expressed in the myocardium, most of the therapeutic drugs for the heart failure target only 2 receptors, β1 adrenergic receptor (β1AR) and angiotensin (Ang) II type 1 receptor (AT1R) [3, 4]. However, the blockers against β1AR and AT1R are not enough for the treatment of heart failure patients. As the heart failure remains a leading cause of death in developed countries, and the development of the epoch-making cure is desired from the viewpoint for improving the quality of life and reducing the medical cost of the patient [4]. GPCRs is certainly one of the promising target molecules for the treatment of the heart failure, and a better understanding of the components that participate in GPCR signaling pathways in healthy and failing hearts may provide a mechanistic basis for improving heart failure treatment.

1. G PROTEIN SIGNALING AND ITS REGULATORS IN THE HEART

The binding of "ligands", including neurotransmitters and hormones, to the extracellular or intramembrane sites of the receptor activates GPCR signaling. Ligand binding induces conformational changes in the GPCR by disrupting the ionic interaction between the third cytoplasmic loop and the sixth transmembrane region and allows for coupling with G proteins [5, 6]. G proteins form heterotrimer comprised of α, β, and γ subunits at the resting state. The activated form of the receptor can catalyze the exchange of GTP for GDP bound to the α subunit (Gα) of specific G protein, leading to dissociation of Gα from $\beta\gamma$ dimmer (G$\beta\gamma$). Both Gα and G$\beta\gamma$ couple with the respective effectors to activate the independent signaling pathways (Figure 1). The Gα has an intrinsic GTPase activity to hydrolyze GTP into GDP, and GTP hydrolysis will terminate the activation of G protein signaling. The conformation switch between GDP-bound state and GTP-bound state is called "G (protein) cycle" [7].

Several modulators of G protein cycling except GPCRs also participate in the regulation of cardiac function. For example, regulator of G protein signaling (RGS) proteins function as GTPase-activating protein (GAP) of G proteins, which promotes the inactivation of G proteins [8]. It is thought that RGS2, a specific RGS for Gα_q, and RGS4, a specific RGS for Gα_q and Gα_i, play an important role in the heart. Pressure overload-induced cardiac hypertrophy is reportedly suppressed in spite of increase in mortality in transgenic mice with cardiomyocyte-specific overexpression of RGS4. In addition, RGS2-deficient mice have been shown to cause increased mortality in response to pressure overload [9, 10]. On the other hand, one of activator of G protein signaling (AGS) families, AGS8, promotes the G$\beta\gamma$-dependent apoptosis signal [11]. Furthermore, nucleoside diphosphate kinase (NDPK), which induces phosphorylation of His^{266} residue of Gβ to form a signal complex with G$\beta\gamma$, promotes Gα_s-mediated cAMP production in a receptor-independent manner, resulting in enhancement of cardiac muscle contractility [12]. Thus, AGS8 and NDPK are thought to activate G protein signaling pathways through inhibition of heterotrimer formation of Gα with G$\beta\gamma$.

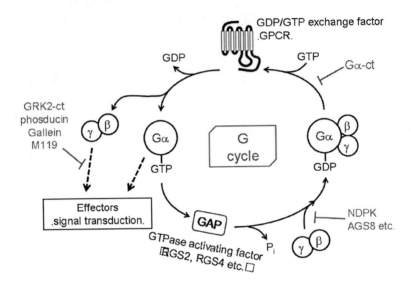

Figure 1. G protein cycle and its regulators

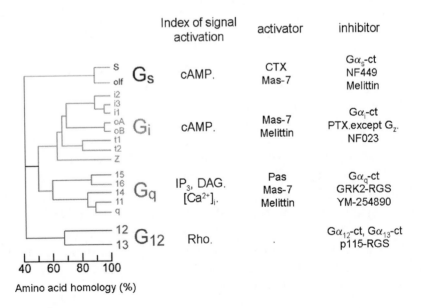

Figure 2. G protein subfamilies and their pharmacological tools. CTX; *Cholera* toxin, Mas-7; mastoparan-7, PTX; pertussis toxin, Pas; *Pasteurella multocida* toxin

2. ASSESSMENT OF G PROTEIN SIGNALING

Multiple G proteins have been identified in all of the eukaryotic organisms. Approximately 20% of the amino acids are found to be conserved from the alignment of deduced amino acid sequences of all the α subunits (Figure 2). G protein is classified into four families (G_s, G_i, G_q, G_{12}) on the basis of amino acid sequence similarity and the functional difference of an effector molecule activated by $G\alpha$. Activation of each G protein signaling can be evaluated by the production of second messenger through activation of its effector enzyme (e.g., $G\alpha_s$ is assessed by activation of adenylyl cyclase, $G\alpha_i$ is by suppression of adenylyl cyclase, and $G\alpha_q$ is by activation of phospholipase C (PLC)). In addition, commercial toxins or reagents which activate or inactivate the specific G protein signaling have become able to easily evaluate the involvement of G protein in various cellular functions. However, a sufficient attention will be required for the interpretation of the results obtained using these toxins, because the purified toxins often contains endotoxins, such as lipopolysaccharide, which may influence the signaling pathways in addition to modification of G proteins. It is also necessary to consider that toxins can bind to membrane proteins to induce cellular responses, which are different from the binding molecules that are required for delivering them into the cytosol. In fact, we recently found that *Pertussis* toxin (PTX), which ADP-ribosylates $G\alpha_i$ and uncouples receptors from G_i, stimulates Toll-like receptor 4 that leads to increase in the number of AT1Rs [13]. In order to overcome these problems, biological approaches to inhibit the function of specific G protein have been conducted. For example, overexpression of each carboxyl-terminal region of $G\alpha$ ($G\alpha$-ct) can induce subtype-specific inhibition of G protein signaling by the competition of corresponding $G\alpha$ to couple with receptors [14, 15]. In addition to $G\alpha$-ct, there is another tool to specifically inhibit $G\alpha$-mediated signaling. An RGS domain polypeptide specifically inhibits $G\alpha$-mediated signaling pathway(s). In contrast to availability of various tools to inhibit $G\alpha$-mediated signaling, there is almost one tool to inhibit $G\beta\gamma$-mediated signaling. A carboxyl-terminal region of G protein-coupled receptor kinase 2 (GRK2-ct, GRK2 is also named as β adrenergic receptor kinase 1 (βARK1)) specifically inhibits $G\beta\gamma$-mediated signaling (Figure 1). More recently, knockdown of specific $G\alpha$ subtype using RNA interference method has been performed to prove the involvement of the specific $G\alpha$.

On the other hand, functional roles of G_{12} family protein (G_{12} and G_{13}; $G_{12/13}$) are hardly analyzed, as $G_{12/13}$ proteins do not participate in the production of second messengers, such as cAMP and Ca^{2+} that can be easily detected, and specific inhibitor of $G_{12/13}$ signaling including a toxin has not been found [16]. $G\alpha_{12/13}$ proteins are a PTX-insensitive G protein found by cloning from mouse brain cDNA library, and are found to be widely expressed in a variety of tissues. Although the $G\alpha_{12}$ knockout (KO) mouse does not show any apparent phenotype, the $G\alpha_{13}$-KO mouse shows embryonic lethality due to lack of angiogenesis [17]. In addition, $G_{12/13}$ proteins are abundantly expressed in platelets, and are shown to couple with $G_{q/11}$ protein-coupled receptors such as thrombin and thromboxane A_2 receptors, those of which can induce platelet aggregation. Both activated $G\alpha_{12}$ and $G\alpha_{13}$ are able to combine with GDP/GTP exchange factor of small G protein Rho (RhoGEF), leading to Rho activation. Results of the study using tissue-specific $G\alpha_{12/13}$-KO mice have shown that $G\alpha_{12/13}$-mediated Rho activation is essential for platelet aggregation and contraction of vascular smooth muscle induced by receptor stimulation [16, 18]. Thus, at least in the present, it is thought that it is the best index to measure Rho activity for evaluating the magnitude of activation of $G\alpha_{12/13}$ signaling.

3. G PROTEINS AND HEART FAILURE

The contraction/relaxation exercise of heart muscle is elegantly regulated by sympathetic and parasympathetic systems. Figure 3 shows the GPCRs expressed in cardiomyocytes and respective GPCR-G protein signaling pathways in the heart. Both β1 and β2 adrenergic receptors (β1AR and β2AR) and adenosine receptor type A2 (A2R) are G_s protein-coupled receptors, and stimulation of these receptors can induce inotropic and chronotropic effects of the myocardium [19, 20]. Activation of G_s-coupled receptors induces activation of protein kinase A (PKA), Epac, and cyclic nucleotide-gated cation (CNG) channels through $G\alpha_s$-mediated cAMP production, and activation of β-arrestin-dependent signaling pathways, including desensitization and downregulation of receptors, through Gβγ-mediated activation of GRK2. Muscarinic acetylcholine (Ach) receptor type 2 (M2R) and A1R are G_i-coupled receptors, and stimulation of these receptors can induce negative chronotropic effect of myocardium through inhibition of L-type Ca^{2+} channel (LTCC) by inhibition of adenylyl cyclase and Gβγ-mediated activation of I_{KAch}

K^+ channels (GIRK). Results of the studies using transgenic (Tg) and KO mice have revealed that G_s protein participates in positive inotropic and chronotropic effects induced by βAR stimulation and $G_{i/o}$ proteins participate in a negative chronotropic effect induced by muscarinic M2 receptor stimulation (Table 1). On the other hand, it is thought that sympathetic nerve system and rennin-Ang II-aldosterone system play a pivotal role in the development of heart failure. These neurohumoral factors induce structural changes of the heart (remodeling) and cardiac dysfunction through activation of G_q and $G_{12/13}$ signaling pathways. Here, we will introduce recent findings including our works about pathophysiological role of each G protein family in heart failure.

3.1. G_s Family Protein and Cardiac Apoptosis

The G_s family protein mainly regulates myocardial contraction through adenylyl cyclase-mediated cAMP production. Persistent activation of $G\alpha_s$ signaling pathway induces cardiomyocyte hypertrophy and accumulation of extracellular matrix proteins (fibrosis), resulting in heart failure [21]. Although $G\alpha_s$-knockout mice exhibits early embryonic lethality [22], transgenic mice with cardiomyocyte-specific overexpression of $G\alpha_s$ show remarkable increase in heart rate and left ventricular contractility induced by catecholamine stimulation, but these mice eventually show cardiac dysfunction accompanying myocardial apoptosis [23]. This mechanism is partly explained that the protein kinase A-mediated excessive phosphorylation of ryanodine receptor type 2 (RyR2) causes increase in Ca^{2+} leak from sarcoplasmic reticulum. In addition, calmodulin (CaM)-dependent kinase II (CaMKII) has been implicated in myocardium apoptosis induced by β1AR stimulation [19]. The mechanism of CaMKII activation includes Ca^{2+}/CaM-dependent pathway induced by the increase in intracellular Ca^{2+} concentration ($[Ca^{2+}]_i$) and a Ca^{2+}-independent pathway caused by the methionine oxidation, and the Ca^{2+}-dependent CaMKII activation pathway appears to participate in $G\alpha_s$-mediated myocardial dysfunction [24].

3.2. Gi Family Protein and Cardioprotection

The $G\alpha_{i/o}$ proteins have been demonstrated to be increased in expression level as well as activity in patients with heart failure [25]. As the $G\alpha_{i2}$ promoter contains a cAMP-responsive CCAAT box, increased sympathetic drive in the failing heart is essential for the proposed mechanism of $G\alpha_{i/o}$ upregulation in heart failure, and the $G\alpha_{i/o}$ upregulation seems to be an apparent negative-feedback response to excess βAR-$G\alpha_s$ signaling. However, treatment with βAR blockers or Ang-converting enzyme inhibitors hardly abolishes G_i upregulation, even though these drugs normalize the plasma concentration levels of catecholamine. Thus, it has not been yet established whether the functional significance of $G\alpha_{i/o}$ upregulation is adaptive or maladaptive response of the heart. It has been recently reported that myocardial cell death induced by ischemia/reperfusion is enhanced in transgenic mice with cardiomyocyte-specific overexpression of $G\alpha_{i2}$-specific inhibitory polypeptide ($G\alpha_{i2}$-ct) [26].

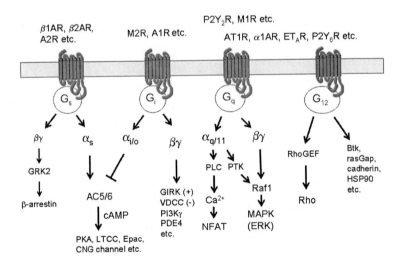

Figure 3. G protein-coupled receptors expressing in the heart. AC; adenylyl cyclase, GIRK; G protein-activated inwardly rectifying K^+ channel, LTCC; L-type Ca^{2+} channel, PDE; phosphodiesterase, PTK; protein tyrosine kinase, VDCC; voltage-dependent Ca^{2+} channels (P/Q-type, N-type)

We have also reported that treatment of rat cardiomyocytes with high concentration of hydrogen peroxide induces $G\alpha_{i/o}$ activation and consequent

G$\beta\gamma$ released from G$\alpha_{i/o}$ induces activation of survival factors such as Akt and extracellular signal-regulated kinase (ERK) through phosphatidylinositol-3-kinase (PI3K), and that functional inhibition of G$\beta\gamma$ signaling by the expression of GRK2-ct enhances myocardium cell death caused by oxidative stress [27]. In addition, tachycardia-induced cardiomyopathy is suppressed in transgenic mice with cardiomyocyte-specific expression of a constitutively active mutant of Gα_{i2} (CA-Gα_{i2}) [28]. Taken together, the G$_i$ family protein signaling may work on protection of the heart from various stresses.

3.3. G$_q$ Family Protein and Hypertrophy

From a variety of evidence using genetically modified mice with cardiomyocyte-specific overexpression or disruption of G$_q$ family proteins or their regulatory proteins, the G$\alpha_{q/11}$-mediated signaling pathway plays a pivotal role in the development of cardiac hypertrophy [29-32]. Several G$_q$ protein-coupled receptor agonists, such as Ang II, endothelin (ET)-1, and norepinephrine, is known to induce hypertrophic gene expression through Ca^{2+}-dependent signaling pathways. About 10 years ago, the mechanism of Ca^{2+}-mediated hypertrophy was first proposed by Molkentin *et al.* that Ca^{2+}-dependent transcription factor, nuclear factor of activated T cells (NFAT), mediates G$\alpha_{q/11}$-mediated cardiac hypertrophy through increases in $[Ca^{2+}]_i$ [33]. Although a variety of evidence using transgenic and knockout mice have suggested that Gα_q-mediated Ca^{2+} signaling pathway plays a central role in the development of hypertrophy, it is still unclear how Gα_q-mediated signaling specifically encodes the alteration of intracellular Ca^{2+} concentration ($[Ca^{2+}]_i$) on the background of the rhythmic Ca^{2+} increases required for contraction.

In non-excitable cells, it is generally thought that inositol-1,4,5-trisphosphate (IP$_3$) produced by PLC-mediated hydrolysis of phosphatidylinositol-4,5-bisphosphate predominantly regulates agonist-induced Ca^{2+} signaling. However, we found that diacylglycerol (DAG), but not IP$_3$, mediates agonist-induced sustained Ca^{2+} signaling in excitable cardiomyocytes [34]. The DAG-mediated cation influx is essential for agonist-induced membrane depolarization, and the activation of voltage-dependent Ca^{2+} channels via increase in resting potential mainly contributes to agonist-induced Ca^{2+} influx required for cardiomyocyte hypertrophy (Figure 4).

Table 1. Results of functional analyses using genetic mutated mice

Reference	target protein	phenotype	Results of functional analysis
Iwase M et al (1996) Iwase M et al (1997)	Gα$_s$ (short form)-Tg*	cardiomyopathy with aging	enhancement of response to catecholamine enhancement of induction of cardiac apoptosis
Yu S et al (1998)	Gα$_s$-KO	early embryonic lethal	
Rudolph U et al (1995) [56]	Gα$_{i2}$-KO	inflammatory bowel disease with increase in T$_H$-1 type cytokines	die within a few days after birth by β2AR overexpression in cardiomyocytes (Foerster K et al, 2003 [53]), ablation of LTCC inhibition inducedby M2R stimulation in atrial myocytes (Chen F et al, 2001[54]; Nagata K et al, 2000 [55])
Valenzuela D et al (1997) [57]	Gα$_o$-KO	growth retardation, impaired postnatal survival	
Zhu M et al (2008)	CA-Gα$_{o1}$-Tg	normal development, survival rate and cardiac shape	enhancement of Ca^{2+} handling and LV systolic function due to PP2A suppression
Bauer A et al (2008)	CA-Gα$_{i2}$-Tg	decrease in LV systolic function and heart rate	prevention of tachycardia-induced cardiomyopathy
DeGeorge BR Jr et al (2008)	Gα$_{i2}$-ct-Tg	normal development, survival rate and cardiac shape	increase in cardiac apoptosis induced by ischemia/reperfusion, deteriolation of cardiac dysfunction after myocardial infarction
Williams ML et al (2004)	βARK-ct-Tg	enhancement of β1AR signaling due to inhibition of β1AR desensitization	prevention of cardiac dysfunction caused by pressure overload or myocardial infarction
D'Angelo DD et	WT or CA-Gα$_q$-	cardiac hypertrophy, heart	increase in caspase-dependent myocardial

al (1997)	Tg	failure, increase in mortality	apoptosis induced by pressure overload (Hayakawa Y et al, 2003 [58])
Rogers JH et al (1999)	RGS4-Tg	normal development, survival rate and cardiac shape	increase in mortality induced by pressure overload, suppresion of pressure overload-induced cardiac hypertrophy
Akhter SA et al (1998)	$G\alpha_q$-ct	normal development, survival rate and cardiac shape	suppression of pressure overload-induced cardiac hypertrophy
Offermanns et al (1998)	$G\alpha_q/G\alpha_{11}$-KO	embryonic lethal	embryonic lethal due to myocardial hypoplasia, craniofacial abnormalities
Wettschureck N et al (2001)	$G\alpha_{q/11}$-CKO	normal development, survival rate and cardiac shape	suppression of pressure overload-induced cardiac hypertrophy
Takimoto E et al (2009)	RGS2-KO	normal development, survival rate and cardiac shape	enhancement of $G\alpha_q$-mediated hypertrophy, failure and sudden death induced by pressure overload
Nishida et al (2008)	CA–$G\alpha_{13}$-Tg	normal development, survival rate and cardiac shape	interstitial fibrosis without myocardial hypertrophy, mild LV diastolic dysfunction
Nishida et al (2008)	p115-RGS-Tg	normal development, survival rate and cardiac shape	suppression of cardiac fibrosis and LV dysfunction induced by pressure overload

Tg, cardiomyocyte-specific transgenic mice; KO, knockout mice; CKO, cardiomyocyte-specific conditional knockout mice, CA, constitutively active; LTCC, L-type Ca2+ channel; □AR, □ adrenergic receptor; M2R, muscarinic acetylcholine receptor type 2; LV, left ventricular; PP1, protein phosphatase 1.

Transient receptor potential canonical (TRPC) subfamily channels are putative molecular candidate for receptor-activated cation channels [35]. We found that DAG-activated TRPC channels (TRPC3 and TRPC6) work as key mediators in agonist-induced cardiomyocyte hypertrophy [34]. This finding is supported by the recent report that cardiomyocyte-specific overexpression of diacylglycerol kinase ε, a degrading enzyme of DAG, restores cardiac dysfunction induced by pressure overload in mice [36]. Furthermore, we recently reported that chronic treatment with a novel TRPC3-selective inhibitor after surgical transverse aortic constriction attenuates pressure overload-induced cardiac hypertrophy *in vivo* [37]. In contrast, it has been recently reported that DAG-insensitive TRPC1 channel also participates in pressure overload-induced cardiac hypertrophy *in vivo* [38]. As TRPC1 is also known to function as a scaffold protein to form a signal complex [35], TRPC1, TRPC3 and C6 proteins may assemble to form DAG-activated cation channels, which mediate the $G\alpha_q$-induced cardiac hypertrophy (Figure 4).

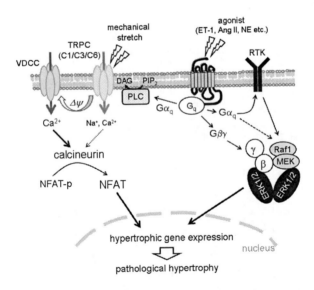

Figure 4. Hypothetical mechanism of G_q-mediated cardiac hypertrophy. VDCC; voltage-dependent Ca^{2+} channels (L-type, T-type), RTK; receptor tyrosine kinase

These results strongly suggest that DAG-activated TRPC channels function as key mediators in $G\alpha_q$-mediated cardiac hypertrophy, and that DAG-activated TRPC channels are potential therapeutic targets for the treatment of heart failure. Although G_q protein-coupled purinergic $P2Y_2$ receptor ($P2Y_2R$) and muscarinic M1 receptor (M1R) are also expressed in rat cardiomyocytes (Figure 3), and we have confirmed that treatment with ATP and Ach induce oscillatory Ca^{2+} response in rat neonatal cardiomyocytes (unpublished data), ATP and Ach do not induce cardiomyocyte hypertrophy [39, 40]. The mechanism is still unknown.

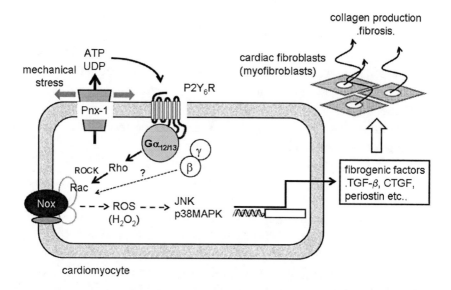

Figure 5. Hypothetical mechanism of $G_{12/13}$-mediated cardiac fibrosis induced by pressure overload. Pnx-1; pannexin-1, H_2O_2; hydrogen peroxide, Nox; NADPH oxidase

The extracellular signal-regulated kinase (ERK) has been also implicated in G_q family protein-mediated cardiac hypertrophy. An interesting work concerned about the molecular mechanism underlying G_q-mediated ERK activation has been recently reported [41]. They have shown that $G\beta\gamma$ released from $G\alpha_q$ upon G_q-coupled receptor stimulation forms a signal complex with ERK1/2 dimer, leading to autophosphorylation of ERK1/2 at Thr^{188} residue and subsequent nuclear localization of ERK1/2, resulting in induction of hypertrophic gene expression. The $G\beta\gamma$ derived from $G\alpha_{i/o}$ proteins upon G_i-coupled receptor stimulation is unable to induce autophosphorylation of ERK1/2. They also show that suppression of ERK1/2 autophosphorylation completely suppressed pressure overload-induced cardiac hypertrophy in mice. This finding accords with the other report that myocardial dysfunction caused by various stresses is improved in mice with cardiomyocyte-specific overexpression of Gβγ-inhibitory peptide (GRK2-ct: βARK-ct) [42, 43].

3.4. G_{12} Family Protein and Cardiac Fibrosis

As shown in figure 3, activation of G_{12} family proteins can induce various effector proteins, including RhoGEF, Bruton's tyrosine kinase (Btk), rasGAP, heat shock protein 90 (HSP90), and rasGAP, in a variety of cell types [44]. However, the study of $G_{12/13}$ protein-mediated signaling in the heart was not performed. Using adenoviral gene transfer method to express $G\alpha_{12/13}$-specifc inhibitory polypeptide, we found that $G_{12/13}$ proteins can be activated by the stimulation of AT1R, ET-1 type A receptor (ET_AR), or α1 adrenergic receptor (α1AR) in primary cultured rat neonatal cardiomyocytes [14, 15, 45]. These are G_q protein-coupled receptors responsible for cardiac hypertrophy, and the hypertrophic responses of cardiomyocytes induced by receptor stimulation are suppressed not only by $G\alpha_q$-specific inhibitory polypeptide but also $G\alpha_{12/13}$-specific inhibitory polypeptide (p115-RGS). Activation of $G\alpha_{12/13}$ by receptor stimulation induces activation of small G protein Rac through activation of Rho and Rho-associated coiled-coil-containing protein kinase (ROCK). In addition, Rac mediates agonist-induced generation of reactive oxygen species (ROS) through NADPH oxidation activation, and generated ROS subsequently activate c-Jun NH_2-terminal kinase (JNK) and p38MAPK [45]. As NADPH oxidase is the only enzyme found in the downstream of the $G\alpha_{12/13}$ proteins and the other three G proteins (G_s, G_i, G_q) activate intracellular signaling pathways through enzymatic production of respective second messengers, ROS may work as a second messenger of the $G_{12/13}$ protein signaling (Figure 5). (deleted: considering that).

Based on the studies using rat cardiomyocytes, we generated a transgenic mice with cardiomyocyte-specific overexpression of p115-RGS (p115-RGS-Tg) and examined whether $G\alpha_{12/13}$ signaling actually participate in cardiac hypertrophy *in vivo*. Surprisingly, we found that pressure overload-induced cardiac hypertrophy was not suppressed, but the interstitial fibrosis and left ventricular diastolic functions were significantly attenuated by the inhibition of myocardial $G\alpha_{12/13}$ signaling [46]. On the contrary, transgenic mice with cardiomyocyte-specific overexpression of constitutively active mutant of $G\alpha_{13}$ (CA-$G\alpha_{13}$) have been shown to cause interstitial fibrosis without accompanying cardiomyocyte hypertrophy. These results suggest that mechanism underlying *in vitro* hypertrophy induced by GPCR stimulation is different from that underlying pressure overload-induced cardiac hypertrophy *in vivo*. The pressure overload-induced activation of Rho, Rac, JNK and p38MAPK, and increase in the expression levels of fibrogenic factors, including transforming growth factor (TGF)-β, periostin, and connective tissue growth factor (CTGF) were remarkably suppressed in p115-RGS-Tg mice. In addition, we found that mechanical stretch-induced ATP release through pannexin-1 hemichannel induces Rho activation in cardiomyocytes and that purinergic P2Y$_6$ receptor-G$\alpha_{12/13}$ signaling in cardiomyocytes triggers pressure overload-induced cardiac fibrosis. Although cardiac fibrosis is believed to accompany with Gα_q-mediated pathological hypertrophy that eventually results in heart failure, our results clearly show that cardiac fibrosis and hypertrophy are independent processes. Furthermore, as pannexin-1 and P2Y$_6$R mRNAs in the heart are upregulated by pressure overload, G$\alpha_{12/13}$-mediated signaling leading to cardiac fibrosis may turn on after myocardial hypertrophy. (deleted: it is speculated that)

4. FUTURE PERSPECTIVES

The G protein signaling of the heart still has many mysteries. For example, cardiomyocyte-specific G$\alpha_{i/o}$-transgenic mice have been reported to show unexpected phenotype that cannot be explained only by the suppression of adenylyl cyclase, suggesting the importance of another effector molecule coupling with G$\alpha_{i/o}$ [47, 48]. In addition, although G proteins have been thought to combine with the effector molecule near the plasma membrane, yeast G protein (Gpa1) is recently shown to couple with an endosome-localized effector molecule PI3K, composed of four subunits including a catalytic subunit Vsp34 and a regulatory subunit Vps15, regulating pheromone response [49]. Also in mammalian cells, it has been reported that intracellular localization and binding affinity to common effector protein of Gα_{12} are different from those of Gα_{13}, and that Gα_i combines with Goloco domain of Pins/Insc at the apical cortex to form signal complex, maintaining cell polarity to regulate asymmetric cell division and spindle-cortex interactions [50, 51]. These findings provide the possibility that localization of G protein regulates the function of cardiomyocytes in a receptor-independent manner.

After the relationship between cardiac fibrosis and left ventricular diastolic dysfunction has been shown, functions of cardiac fibroblasts have been increasingly focused [52]. The roles of G protein signaling in cardiac fibroblasts are studied mainly using primary culture cells. However, the roles of G protein signaling in cardiac fibroblasts have not been well understood *in vivo*, as the promoter gene specific for cardiac fibroblasts is not so far identified. Thus, in order to distinguish the role of G protein signaling in cardiac fibroblasts from that in cardiomyocytes *in vivo*, it will be necessary to use transgenic expression of Gα protein in cardiac fibroblasts, conditional-KO mice with cardiac fibroblast-specific deletion of Gα protein, or conventional Gα-KO mice cross-fertilized with cardiac fibroblast-specific Gα transgenic mice.

5. CONCLUSION

Using a genetically engineered mouse, the G protein signaling responsible for the development of heart failure has been gradually elucidated. Future studies using cardiomyocyte-specific conditional KO mice will provide understanding of the pathophysiological roles of G protein signaling in cardiomyocytes and non-myocytes, respectively. Constructing pharmacological tools for analyzing G protein signaling pathway, we identified new therapeutic targets (TRPC3/TRPC6 channels, P2Y$_6$ receptor) for the treatment of heart failure. Further studies using conditional KO mice will establish the importance of these proteins in heart failure.

REFERENCES

[1]   Gudermann, T., Nurnberg, B. & Schultz, G. (1995). Receptors and G proteins are primary components of transmembrane signal transduction. Part 1. G-protein-coupled receptors: structure and function. *J Mol Med.*, *73*, 51-63.

[2]   Fitzgibbons, T. P., Meyer, T. E. & Aurigemma, G. P. (2009). Mortality in diastolic heart failure: an update. *Cardiol Rev.*, *17*, 51-55.

[3]   Tang, C. M. & Insel, P. A. (2004). GPCR expression in the heart; "new" receptors in myocytes and fibroblasts. *Trends Cardiovas Med*, *14*, 94-99.

[4]   Hunt, S. A., Abraham, W. T., Chin, M. H., Feldman, A. M., Francis, G. S., Ganiats, T. G., Jessup, M., Konstam, M. A., Mancini, D. M., Michl, K., Oates, J. A., Rahko, P. S., Silver, M. A., Stevenson, L. W., Yancy, C.

W., Antman, E. M., Smith, S. C. Jr., Adams, C. D., Anderson, J. L., Faxon, D. P., Fuster, V., Halperin, J. L., Hiratzka, L. F., Jacobs, A. K., Nishimura, R., Ornato, J. P., Page, R. L. & Riegel, B. (2005). ACC/AHA 2005 Guideline Update for the Diagnosis and Management of Chronic Heart Failure in the Adult: a report of the American College of Cardiology/American Heart Association Task Force on Practice Guidelines (Writing Committee to Update the 2001 Guidelines for the Evaluation and Management of Heart Failure): developed in collaboration with the American College of Chest Physicians and the International Society for Heart and Lung Transplantation: endorsed by the Heart Rhythm Society. *Circulation*, *112*, e154-235.

[5]   Gether, U. & Kobilka, B. K. (1998). G protein-coupled receptors. II. Mechanism of agonist activation. *J Biol Chem.*, *273*, 17979-17982.

[6]   Wess, J. (1997). G-protein-coupled receptors: molecular mechanisms involved in receptor activation and selectivity of G-protein recognition. *FASEB J*, *11*, 346-354.

[7]   Simon, M. I., Strathmann, M. P. & Gautam, N. (1991). Diversity of G proteins in signal transduction. *Science*, *252*, 802-808.

[8]   Riddle, E. L., Schwartzman, R. A., Bond, M. & Insel, P. (2005). Multi-tasking RGS proteins in the heart. *Circ Res.*, *96*, 401-411.

[9]   Rogers, J. H., Tamirisa, P., Kovacs, A., Weinheimer, C., Courtois, M., Blumer, K. J., Kelly, D. P. & Muslin, A. J. (1999). RGS4 causes increased mortality and reduced cardiac hypertrophy in response to pressure overload. *J Clin Invest*, *104*, 567-576.

[10]   Takimoto, E., Koitabashi, N., Hsu, S., Ketner, E. A., Zhang, M., Nagayama, T., Bedja, D., Gabrielson, K. L., Blanton, R., Siderovski, D. P., Mendelsohn, M. E. & Kass, D. A. (2009). Regulator of G protein signaling 2 mediates cardiac compensation to pressure overload and antihypertrophic effects of PDE5 inhibition in mice. *J Clin Invest*, *119*, 408-420.

[11]   Sato, M., Cismowski, M. J., Toyota, E., Smrcka, A. V., Lucchesi, P. A., Chilian, W. M. & Lanier, S. M. (2006). Identification of a receptor-independent activator of G protein signaling (AGS8) in ischemic heart and its interaction with Gβγ. *Proc Natl Acad Sci USA*, *103*, 797-802.

[12]   Hippe, H. J., Luedde, M., Lutz, S., Koehler, H., Eschenhagen, T., Frey, N., Katus, H. A., Wieland, T. & Niroomand, F. (2007). Regulation of cardiac cAMP synthesis and contractility by nucleoside diphosphate kinase B/G protein bg dimer complexes. *Circ Res.*, *100*, 1191-1199.

[13] Nishida, M., Suda, M., Tanabe, S., Onohara, N., Nakaya, M., Kanaho, Y., Sumimoto, H., Sato, Y. & Kurose, H. *Pertussis* toxin upregulates angiotensin type 1 receptors through TLR4-mediated Rac activation. JBC, under revision.

[14] Maruyama, Y., Nishida, M., Sugimoto, Y., Tanabe, S., Turner, J.H., Kozasa, T., Wada, T., Nagao, T. & Kurose, H. (2002). G$\alpha_{12/13}$ mediate α1-adrenergic receptor-induced cardiac hypertrophy. *Circ Res.*, *91*, 961-969.

[15] Arai, K., Maruyama, Y., Nishida, M., Tanabe, S., Kozasa, T., Mori, Y., Nagao, T. & Kurose, H. (2003). Differential requirement of Gα_{12}, Gα_{13}, Gα_q, and G$\beta\gamma$ for endothelin-1-induced c-Jun NH$_2$-terminal kinase and extracellular signal-regulated kinase activation. *Mol Pharmacol*, *63*, 478-488.

[16] Wettschureck, N. & Offermanns, S. (2005). Mammalian G proteins and their cell type specific functions. *Physiol Rev.*, *85*, 1159-1204.

[17] Offermanns, S., Macino, V., Revel, J. P. & Simon, M. I. (1997). Vascular system defects and impaired cell chemokinasis as a result of Gα_{13} deficiency. *Scicence*, *275*, 533-536.

[18] Wirth, A., Benyó, Z., Lukasova, M., Leutgeb, B., Wettschureck, N., Gorbey, S., Örsy, P., Horváth, B., Maser-Gluth, C., Greiner, E., Lemmer, B., Schütz, G., Gutkind, J. S. & Offermanns, S. (2008). G$_{12}$-G$_{13}$-LARG-mediated signaling in vascular smooth muscle is required for salt-induced hypertension. *Nat Med*, *14*, 64-68.

[19] Salazar, N. C., Chen, J. & Rockman, H. A. (2007). Cardiac GPCRs: GPCR signaling in healthy and failing hearts. *Biochem Biophys Acta*, *1768*, 1006-1018.

[20] Liang, B. T. & Morley, J. F. (1996). A new cyclic AMP-independent, Gs-mediated stimulatory mechanism via the adenosine A2a receptor in the intact cardiac cell. *J Biol Chem.*, *271*, 18678-18685.

[21] Iwase, M., Bishop, S. P., Uechi, M., Vatner, D. E., Shannon, R. P., Kudej, R. K., Wight, D. C., Wagner, T. E., Ishikawa, Y., Homcy, C. J. & Vatner, S. F. (1996). Adverse effects of chronic endogenous sympathetic drive induced by cardiac Gsα overexpression. *Circ Res.*, *78*, 517-524.

[22] Yu, S., Yu, D., Lee, E., Eckhaus, M., Lee, R., Corria, Z., Accili, D., Westphal, H. & Weinstein, L. S. (1998). Variable and tissue-specific hormone resistance in heterotrimeric G$_s$ protein α-subunit (Gsα) knockout mice is due to tissue-specific imprinting of the Gsα gene. *Proc Natl Acad Sci USA*, *95*, 8715-8720.

[23] Iwase, M., Uechi, M., Vatner, D. E., Asai, K., Shannon, R. P., Kudej, R. K., Wagner, T. E., Wight, D. C., Patrick, T. A., Ishikawa, Y., Homcy, C. J. & Vatner, S. F. (1997). Cardiomyopathy induced by cardiac Gsα overexpression. *Am J Physiol Heart Circ Physiol*, *272*, H585-H589.

[24] Erickson, J. R., Joiner, M. L., Guan, X., Kutschke, W., Yang, J., Oddis, C. V., Bartlett, R. K., Lowe, J. S., O'Donnell, S. E., Aykin-Burns, N., Zimmerman, M. C., Zimmerman, K., Ham, A. J., Weiss, R. M., Spitz, D. R., Shea, M. A., Colbran, R. J., Mohler, P. J. & Anderson, M. E. (2008). A dynamic pathway for calcium-independent activation of CaMKII by methionine oxidation. *Cell*, *133*, 462-474.

[25] Feldman, A. M., Cates, A. E., Veazey, W. B., Hershberger, R. E., Bristow, M. R., Baughman, K. L., Baumgartner, W. A. & Van Dop, C. (1988). Increase of the 40,000-mol wt pertussis toxin substrate (G protein) in the failing human heart. *J Clin Invest*, *82*, 189-197.

[26] DeGeorge, B. R. Jr., Gao, E., Boucher, M., Vinge, L. E., Martini, J. S., Raake, P. W., Chuprun, J. K., Harris, D. M., Kim, G. W., Soltys, S., Eckhart, A. D. & Koch, W. J. (2008). Targeted inhibition of cardiomyocyte Gi signaling enhances susceptibility to apoptotic cell death in response to ischemic stress. *Circulation*, *117*, 1378-1387.

[27] Nishida, M., Maruyama, Y., Tanaka, R., Kontani, K., Nagao, T. & Kurose, H. (2000). Gα$_i$ and Gα$_o$ are target proteins of reactive oxygen species. *Nature*, *408*, 492-495.

[28] Bauer, A., McDonald, A. D., Nasir, K., Peller, L., Rade, J. J., Miller, J. M., Heldman, A. W. & Donahue, J. K. (2004). Inhibitory G protein overexpression provides physiologically relevant heart rate control in persistent atrial fibrillation. *Circulation*, *110*, 3115-3120.

[29] D'Angelo, D. D., Sakata, Y., Lorenz, J. N., Boivin, G. P., Walsh, R. A., Liggett, S. B. & Dorn, G. W. 2nd. (1997). Transgenic Gα$_q$ overexpression induces cardiac contractile failure in mice. *Proc Natl Acad Sci USA*, *94*, 8121-8126.

[30] Akhter, S. A., Luttrell, L. M., Rockman, H. A., Iaccarino, G., Lefkowitz, R. J. & Koch, W. J. (1998). Targeting the receptor-G$_q$ interface to inhibit *in vivo* pressure overload myocardial hypertrophy. *Science*, *280*, 574-577.

[31] Offermanns, S., Zhao, L. P., Gohla, A., Sarosi, I., Simon, M. I. & Wilkie, T. M. (1998). Embryonic cardiomyocyte hypoplasia and craniofacial defects in Gα$_q$/Gα$_{11}$-mutant mice. *EMBO J*, *17*, 4304-4312.

[32] Wettschureck, N., Rutten, H., Zywietz, A., Gehring, D., Wilkie, T. M., Chen, J., Chien, K. R. & Offermanns, S. (2001). Absence of pressure

overload induced myocardial hypertrophy after conditional inactivation of $G\alpha_q/G\alpha_{11}$ in cardiomyocytes. *Nat Med.*, 7, 1236-1240.

[33] Molkentin, J. D., Lu, J. R., Antos, C. L., Markham, B., Richardson, J., Robbins, J., Grant, S. R. & Olson, E. N. (1998). A calcineurin-dependent transcriptional pathway for cardiac hypertrophy. *Cell*, *93*, 215-228.

[34] Onohara, N., Nishida, M., Inoue, R., Kobayashi, H., Sumimoto, H., Sato, Y., Mori,Y., Nagao, T. & Kurose, H. (2006). TRPC3 and TRPC6 are essential for angiotensin II-induced cardiac hypertrophy. *EMBO J*, *25*, 5305-5316.

[35] Nishida, M. & Kurose, H. (2008). Roles of TRP channels in the development of cardiac hypertrophy. *Naunyn Schmiedebergs Arch Pharmacol*, *378*, 395-406.

[36] Niizeki, T., Takeishi, Y., Kitahara, T., Arimoto, T., Ishino, M., Bilim, O., Suzuki, S., Sasaki, T., Nakajima, O., Walsh, R. A., Goto, K. & Kubota, I. (2008). Diacylglycerol kinase-epsilon restores cardiac dysfunction under chronic pressure overload: a new specific regulator of $G\alpha_q$ signaling cascade. *Am J Physiol Heart Circ Physiol*, *295*, H245-H255.

[37] Kiyonaka, S., Kato, K., Nishida, M., Mio, K., Numaga, T., Sawaguchi, Y., Yoshida, T., Wakamori, M., Mori, E., Numata, T., Ishii, M., Takemoto, H., Ojida, A., Watanabe, K., Uemura, A., Kurose, H., Morii, T., Kobayashi, T., Sato, Y., Sato, C., Hamachi, I. & Mori, Y. (2009). Selective and direct inhibition of TRPC3 channels underlies biological activities of a pyrazole compound. *Proc Natl Acad Sci USA*, *106*, 5400-5405.

[38] Seth, M., Zhang, Z. S., Mao, L., Graham, V., Burch, J., Stiber, J., Tsiokas, L., Winn, M., Abramowitz, J., Rockman, H. A., Birnbaumer, L. & Rosenberg, P. (2009). TRPC1 channels are critical for hypertrophic signaling in the heart. *Circ Res*, *105*, 1023-1030.

[39] Post, G. R., Goldstein, D., Thuerauf, D. J., Glembotski, C. C. & Brown, J. H. (1996). Dissociation of p44 and p42 mitogen-activated protein kinase activation from receptor-induced hypertrophy in neonatal rat ventricular myocytes. *J Biol Chem.*, *271*, 8452-8457.

[40] Pham, T. M., Morris, J. B., Arthur, J. F., Post, G. R., Brown, J. H. & Woodcock, E. A. (2003). UTP but not ATP causes hypertrophic growth in neonatal rat cardiomyocytes. *J Mol Cell Cardiol*, *35*, 287-292.

[41] Lorentz, K., Schmitt, J. P., Schmitteckert, E. M. & Lohse, M. J. (2009). A new type of ERK1/2 autophosphorylation causes cardiac hypertrophy. *Nat Med*, *15*, 75-83.

[42] Rockman, H. A., Chien, K. R., Choi, D. J., Iaccarino, G., Hunter, J. J., Ross, J. J., Lefkowitz, R. & Koch, W. J. (1998). Expression of a β-adrenergic receptor kinase 1 inhibitor prevents the development of myocardial failure in gene-targeted mice. *Proc Natl Acad Sci USA, 95,* 7000-7005.

[43] Williams, M. L., Hata, J. A., Schroder, J., Rampersaud, E., Petrofski, J., Jakoi, A., Milano, C. A. & Koch, W. J. (2004). Targeted beta-adrenergic receptor kinase (betaARK1) inhibition by gene transfer in failing human hearts. *Circulation, 109,* 1590-1593.

[44] Kurose, H. (2003). Gα12 and Gα13 as key regulatory mediator in signal transduction. *Life Sci., 74,* 155-161.

[45] Nishida, M., Tanabe, S., Maruyama, Y., Mangmool, S., Urayama, K., Nagamatsu, Y., Takagahara, S., Turner, J. H., Kozasa, T., Kobayashi, H., Sato, Y., Kawanishi, T., Inoue, R., Nagao, T. & Kurose, H. (2005). Gα12/13- and reactive oxygen species-dependent activation of c-Jun NH2-terminal kinase and p38 mitogen-activated protein kinase by angiotensin receptor stimulation in rat neonatal cardiomyocytes. *J Biol Chem., 280,* 18434-18441.

[46] Nishida, M., Sato, Y., Uemura, A., Narita, Y., Tozaki-Saitoh, H., Nakaya, M., Ide, T., Suzuki, K., Inoue, K., Nagao, T. & Kurose, H. (2008). P2Y6 receptor-Gα12/13 signalling in cardiomyocytes triggers pressure overload-induced cardiac fibrosis. *EMBO J, 27,* 3104-3115.

[47] Rudolph, U., Finegold, M. J., Rich, S. S., Harriman, G. R., Srinivasan, Y., Brabet, P., Boulay, G., Bradley, A. & Birnbaumer, L. (1995). Ulcerative colitis and adenocarcinoma of the colon in Gαi2-deficient mice. *Nat Genet, 10,* 143-150.

[48] Zhu, M., Gach, A. A., Liu, G., Xu, X., Lim, C. C., Zhang, J. X., Mao, L., Chuprun, K., Koch, W. J., Liao, R., Koren, G., Blaxall, B. C. & Mende, U. (2008). Enhanced calcium cycling and contractile function in transgenic hearts expressing constitutively active Gαo* protein. *Am J Physiol Heart Circ Physiol, 294,* H1335-H1347.

[49] Slessareva, J. E., Routt, S. M., Temple, B., Bankaitis, V. A. & Dohlman, H. G. (2006). Activation of the phosphatidylinositol 3-kinase Vps34 by a G protein α subunit at the endosome. *Cell, 126,* 191-203.

[50] Yamazaki, J., Katoh, H., Yamaguchi, Y. & Negishi, M. (2005). Two G12 family G proteins, Gα12 and Gα13, show different subcellular localization. *Biochem Biophys Res Commun, 332,* 782-786.

[51] Siegrist, S. E. & Doe, C. Q. (2005). Microtubule-induced Pins/Gα_i cortical polarity in *Drosophila* neuroblasts. *Cell, 123*, 1323-1335.

[52] Souders, C. A., Bowers, S. L. & Baudino, T. A. (2009). Cardiac fibroblast: the renaissance cell. *Circ Res., 105*, 1164-1176.

[53] Foerster, K., Groner, F., Matthes, J., Koch, W. J., Birnbaumer, L. & Herzig, S. (2003). Cardioprotection specific for the G protein Gi2 in chronic adrenergic signaling through β2-adrenoceptors. *Proc Natl Acad Sci USA, 100*, 14475-14480.

[54] Chen, F., Spicher, K., Jiang, M., Birnbaumer, L. & Wetzel, G. T. (2001). Lack of muscarinic regulation of Ca^{2+} channels in Gα_{i2} gene knockout mouse hearts. *Am J Physiol Heart Circ Physiol, 280*, H1989-H1995.

[55] Nagata, K., Ye, C., Jain, M., Milstone, D. S., Liao, R. & Mortensen, R. M. (2000). Gα_{i2} but not Gα_{i3} is required for muscarinic inhibition of contractility and calcium currents in adult cardiomyocytes. *Circ Res., 87*, 903-909.

[56] Valenzuela, D., Han, X., Mende, U., Fankhauser, C., Mashimo, H., Huang, P., Pfeffer, J., Neer, E. J. & Fishman, M. C. (1997). Gα_o is necessary for muscarinic regulation of Ca^{2+} channels in mouse heart. *Proc Natl Acad Sci USA, 94*, 1727-1732.

[57] Zhu, M., Gach, A. A., Liu, G., Xu, X., Lim, C. C., Zhang, J. X., Mao, L., Chuprun, K., Koch, W. J., Liao, R., Koren, G., Blaxall, B. C. & Mende, U. (2008). Enhanced calcium cycling and contractile function in transgenic hearts expressing active Gα_o* protein. *Am J Physiol Heart Circ Physiol, 294*, H1335-H1347.

[58] Hayakawa, Y., Chandra, M., Miao, W., Shirani, J., Brown, J. H., Dorn, G. W. 2nd., Armstrong, R. C. & Kitsis, R. N. (2003). Inhibition of cardiac myocyte apoptosis improves cardiac function and abolishes mortality in the peripartum cardiomyopathy of Gα_q transgenic mice. *Circulation, 108*, 3036-3041.

In: Heart Failure: Symptoms, Causes...   ISBN: 978-1-61668-959-9
Editor: Madison S. Wright, pp. 73-87   © 2010 Nova Science Publishers, Inc.

Chapter 4

THE ROLE OF UROTENSIN II IN THE DEVELOPMENT AND MANAGEMENT OF CONGESTIVE HEART FAILURE

*William Noiles and Adel Giaid**

Department of Medicine, McGill University Health Centre, Montreal,
Quebec, Canada

ABSTRACT

Urotensin II (UII) has been shown to cause an endothelium dependant vascular response which has been linked to hypertension and atherosclerosis. It is believed that UII acts on receptors on the intact endothelium to release NO and other vasoactive molecules to cause dilation. In individuals with a damaged endothelium it appears that UII acts directly on VSMC to cause increased contraction via the PKC pathway. More recently UII has been implicated in congestive heart failure, playing a role in cardiac contraction, hypertrophy and collagen deposition. Initial studies in animal models show that the use of UII-antagonists ameliorate the negative responses that occur following

---

* Corresponding author: Cardiology, McGill University Health Centre, 1650 Cedar Avenue, Montreal, Quebec H3G 1C6, Canada, Tel: 514 934 1934 ext: 43841, Fax: 514 934 8448, Email: adel.giaid@mcgill.ca

damage to the heart, further implicating UII as an important mediator of cardiac change and potential therapeutic target.

INTRODUCTION

Urotensin II (UII) is a vasoactive peptide that was originally found in the goby fish, with homologs later found in several other species including mice, rats, frogs and humans [9, 10]. Given its similarity with somatostation it was originally believed that the two might share a common receptor [8]. However Ames et al found that UII was the ligand for its own receptor, the rat orphan GPR14/SENR [1], which in humans is now known as the urotensin II receptor (UTR). As is the case with UII and somatostatin, the UII receptor shares structural similarity with the somatostatin receptor as well as opiod receptors. UII was originally reported to be the most potent vasoconstrictor found to date [1], acting on the UT receptor to mobilize intracellular calcium stores, however it now appears that UII may have drastically different effects depending on the species, cell type and integrity of the endothelium. In humans it appears that UII activity is closely linked to the integrity of the endothelium, acting as a vasodilator in vessels with an intact endothelium but vasoconstrictive in those with dysfunctional endothelium. Disease states linked to the development of congestive heart failure including: hypertension, atherosclerosis, and diabetes, all show increased plasma levels of UII.

Congestive heart failure (CHF) is a condition in which the heart is not able to sufficiently pump blood to the body's organ. It can be classified as systolic, when there is an inability for the heart to contract properly leading to decreased ejection fraction, or diastolic, when decreases in relaxation result in blood to back up, causing pulmonary edema. The increased demand on the heart to maintain function results in increase stress on the muscle, hypertrophy and eventually cell death. Risk factors for CHF include: coronary artery disease, hypertension, atherosclerosis, diabetes, congenital heart defects, and cardiomyopathies. Given the role of several neurohormones in the progression of CHF (rennin-angiotensin, aldosterone, epinephrine, and serotonin to name a few) it is quite possible that UII may also take part. UII has been shown to play a role in the progression of CHF risk factors, indirectly contributing to heart failure. More recently UII has been shown to impact the heart directly, further contributing to the development of this disease.

Urotensin II Mediated Pathology

Hypertension and atherosclerosis

When originally discovered UII was hailed as the most potent vasoconstrictor ever found, acting as such in all vessels tested [1]. However studies of UII in various species have shown varied actions depending on the vessel, species UII was derived from, integrity of the endothelium and the presence or absence of a diseased state [1, 2, 16, 22, 23, 27, 29, 35, 43]. Initial studies by Ames found that UII acts on vessels as a very potent vasoconstrictor [1], however it was soon demonstrated that these effects are not universal. It was later shown that the potency of UII's vasoactive response varies according to vessel group, having a strong vasoconstricting effect in the thoracic aorta and less of a response in the coronary arteries in rabbits [29]. Interestingly they also found that pulmonary arteries, ear arteries and ear veins did not yield any vasoactive response. Further studies have confirmed these varied responses, implying that there must be other factors involved to account for the different vasoactive response induced by UII [23, 27, 35].

In vivo human studies have had even more contradictory findings. Bohm showed that the infusion of human UII lead to constriction of brachial arteries [2] whereas Wilkinson saw, no effects in these vessels upon UII infusion [43]. While the sources of UII differed the more likely explanation for the difference comes from the criteria used to select subjects. Wilkinson's volunteers were older and smokers were excluded from participating. Advanced age and smoking are both associated with an increase prevalence of vascular and cardiovascular problems, meaning these subjects may have underlying pathological differences which may explain the lack of response.

In 2004 Lim and his colleagues set out to find an explanation for the different effects of UII, finding that vasoactivity is dependent on the health of the individual [22]. They had two treatment groups- physiologically healthy individuals and patients with CHF. They discovered that UII actually had vasodilatory effects in healthy individuals whereas patients with CHF showed vessel constriction. It was hypothesized that the physiological role of II may in fact be vasodilatory and vasoconstriction occurs in disease states; earlier studies were mainly done in the absence of an intact endothelium which would account for their findings. The vast differences coming from the various studies highlight an important point: the effects of UII appear to be species specific, and in some cases vessel specific. In fact in stark contrast to the initial findings that UII is the most potent vasoconstrictor, one study actually found that UII is comparable to the most potent vasodilator, adrenomedullin (ADM), in human small pulmonary and abdominal arteries [35]. These varied results show that one cannot generalize on the effects of UII on a particular vasculature bed based on the results used in a different animal model or with UII derived from a different source.

Hypertension has been shown to be the most common risk factor associated with CHF, occurring in as many as 91% of patients in one study and increasing one's risk of developing CHF 2-3 fold [21]. A picture seems to be emerging with UII acting on receptors found on the endothelium of human vessels in physiologically healthy individuals leading to vasodilatation. These effects are proposed to result from the production of NO and other vasoactive molecules by the endothelium in response to UII activation of the endothelial UT receptor [3]. These molecules are then released to act on vessels leading to vasodilatation. In disease states in which there is endothelial dysfunction one sees UII directly stimulating vascular smooth muscle cells (VSMC) resulting in vasoconstriction of vessels [36]. Activation of the UT receptor of VSMC leads to Gq protein activation and the eventual activation of various signal pathways including PLC, which leads to the production of IP_3 and DAG causing the release of Ca^{++} and muscle contraction [24]. Experiments using selective inhibitors of enzymes found in these pathways have attenuated these effects, providing further evidence of UII mediated Ca^{++} release and contraction [31]. However the same study that provided a mechanism for vasoconstriction also showed that human urotensin II caused vasoconstriction in rabbit aorta segments regardless of the state of the endothelium [42]. This finding suggests that UII endothelial activation is not always preferred, meaning the VSMC can be stimulated by UII even in the presence of intact endothelium or that varied vasoactive effects are mediated by different receptor binding, and it is the binding of these alternate receptors that results in different responses. While the endothelium integrity has been shown to play a role in vasoactivity this implies that it is not the only factor determining the response. In fact it is plausible that the vasoactive effects of UII depend on its interaction with other molecules and it is this interaction that decides the vasoactive response in vessels.

Dyslipidaemia leads to increases in LDL cholesterol and mildly oxidized LDL (moxLDL) which subsequently cause the development of atherosclerotic plaques through the stimulation of VSMC differentiation and proliferation. It has been known that moxLDL can interact with vasoactive agents to increase these effects [39], so it is logical to assume that UII, a potent vasoactive agent, may also interact with moxLDL. Indeed studies have shown that UII increases the mitogenic effects of LDL on VSMC in a synergistic manner [40]. These actions are believed to take place via action of the UT G-Protein Coupled Receptor and activation of the cSRC tyrosine kinase- PKC- ERK signalling cascade leading to DNA synthesis in VSMC [42]. UII activates a complimentary pathway with additive effects on proliferation and differentiation of VSMC. These synergistic effects were abolished by the addition of selective inhibitors for c-SRC tyrosine kinase, PKC and ERK, providing further evidence that UII is causing these effects through the activation of this pathway [42].

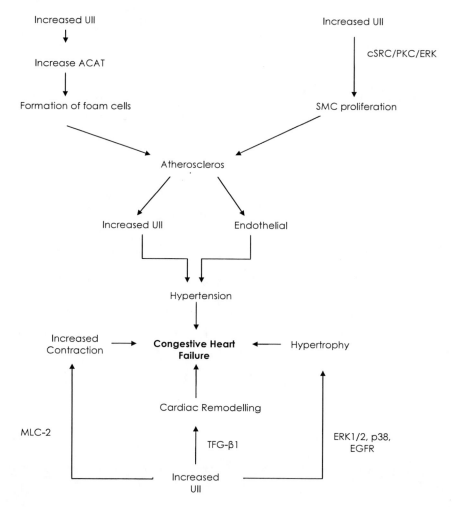

Figure 1.

Table 1. The effects of Human Urotensin II on various vessels in animal models

Species	Vessel	Effect	Notes	Reference
Rat	Thoracic Aorta	Constrictor		Nothacker 1999
	Main Pulmonary Arteries	Constrictor		MacLean 2000
	Small Pulmonary Arteries	None		
Rabbit	Thoracic Aorta	Constrictor		Opgaard 2000
	Coronary Artery	Constrictor (smaller effect)		
	Pulmonary Artery	None		
	Ear Artery	None		
	Ear Vein	None		
Human	Pulmonary Resistance Arteries Abdominal Resistance Arteries	Vasodilate		Stirrat 2001
	Forearm	Constrict	IN VIVO	Bohm 2002
	Brachial Artery	Constrict	IN VIVO	Bohm 2002
		No Effect	IN VIVO	Wilkinson 2002
	Cutaneous vasculator	Dilate normal Constrict CHF		Lim 2004
	Small subcutaneous resistance arteries and veins Internal mammary arteries Saphenous veins	No vasoactivity		Hillier 2001
Non-Human	Left anterior descending	Constrict		Ames 1999

Primates	coronary, left circumflex, mesenteric, pulmonary, renal, proximal descending thoracic aorta, distal descending thoracic aorta, distal abdominal aorta, basilar, common carotid and internal mammary arteries. Portal and jugular veins.		

It is important to note, however, that the effects of UII were partially attenuated by inhibitors of EGF receptor, JNK and ROCK suggesting that the c-SRC/PKC/ERK pathway is not exclusive in its effects on VSMCs. As atherosclerosis develops there is further damage to the vascular endothelium, which is associated with increased negative vasoconstrictive effects of UII [38] contributing to hypertension, a risk factor for atherosclerosis in its own right. UII and UT receptor are upregulated in atherosclerotic lesions [24] further potentiating the progression of UII atherosclerotic damage in a dangerous positive feedback loop.

Atherosclerosis is associated with a build up of cholesterol causing vessel wall thickness and the induction of a chronic inflammatory response that includes the infiltration of monocytes and macrophage. Associated with the progression of atherosclerosis is the development of macrophage derived foam cells. ACAT-1, a protein responsible for the conversion of intracellular cholesterol into lipid droplets which are implicated in plaque formation, has been shown to be crucial for the formation of foam cells [25]. Watanabe et al has shown that ACAT-1 is upregulated in the presence of Urotensin II, resulting in increased production of foam cells in lesions [41]. Also increased in the immune response are lymphocytes, which have been shown to be the largest producers of UII in the body [5]. Thus the initiation of atherosclerosis results in the increased production of UII which then acts to increase differentiation and proliferation of VSMC and foam cell formation causing more endothelial damage. This results in an even greater increase in atherosclerosis of vessels, as well as increases in hypertension induced by UII interactions with a dysfunctional endothelium.

Urotensin II and the Heart

Myocardial UII

UII and its receptor have both been shown to be present in cardiac tissue, however their physiological and pathophysiological roles have yet to be fully determined. Given the detrimental effects of increases in UII in blood vessels during pathology it is likely that increases in the myocardium may play a role in the development of heart failure. The hearts of healthy controls have very low or undetectable levels of UII mRNA and protein, whereas patients with early-stage CHF have weak expression levels, and even greater levels have been observed in patients with end-stage CHF [12]. Important to note is these findings were consistent irrespective of the cause for CHF. Similar results were seen following the induction of a myocardial infarction (MI) in rats [37]. Increased levels of UII and UTR were seen in both the infarct and noninfarct zones of the left ventricle following MI, suggesting a possible pathophysiological role for UII in the heart.

Circulating UII

Several studies have investigated the correlation between plasma and cardiac levels of UII with varied results. It was found that immunoreactive plasma UII was elevated in patients with heart failure, and UII is correlated with endothelin I and adrenomedullin [30]. This was confirmed in another study which also showed that elevated plasma UII occurs regardless of the presence of coronary artery disease [32]. Further it was found that UII levels were higher in the aortic root compared to the pulmonary artery, indicating cardiopulmonary production. Elevated levels of circulating UII were then significantly correlated to functional class and systolic function, suggesting that they may in fact be suitable markers for evaluating CHF [15]. However Dschietzig et al saw no differences in plasma UII and severity of CHF, concluding that the involvement of UII in the development of human CHF is unlikely [13]. Kruger et al found similar results but concluded that hU-II is released and acts locally as opposed to acting as a circulating hormone [18]. It has been suggested that, much like several other neurohormonal systems, UII is upregulated following heart failure as a compensatory mechanism [19]. They also speculate that the possible discrepancies in plasma UII levels may be reflective of differences in assays; suggesting that some groups are detecting bioactive UII whereas others are detecting bioactive UII as well as UII precursors and degradation products. It has been suggested that UII may be a suitable marker for heart failure [26], however further investigation into the correlation between circulating levels of UII and levels in the heart are required before assuming that circulating UII levels may be a good marker for heart failure.

Change in cardiac function

UII has been shown to cause increased contractile force in human atrium and ventricle [34], acting as one of the most potent inotropic agents to date, a finding quite contradictory to a study in monkeys that found contractile dysfunction following UII administration [1]. This stark contrast once again outlines the vast differences in response to UII within different animal models; findings from one study may not be universally applicable to all models. This inotropic response was replicated and it was proposed that hUII causes increased phosphorylation of MLC-2 causing the positive inotropic response [33]. It was also found that hU-II is inversely correlate to left ventricular ejection fraction and positively correlated to left ventricular end diastolic pressure [19].

UII and cardiac hypertrophy

Cardiac hypertrophy is an important step in the development of cardiac failure [20] and as such it is important to determine which neurohormonal factors may play a role in its onset. It has been shown that activation of intracellular protein kinases, particularly mitogen-activated protein kinases (MAPK), lead to the reprogramming of gene expression resulting in increased protein synthesis and hypertrophy [7, 44]. ERKs (members of the MAPK family) were found to be strongly activated by elevated levels of UII in cultured rat cardiomyocytes, indicating dose dependent activation of ERKs following surges in UII levels [45]. Tzanidis et al established an in vitro model using neonatal cardiomyocytes with increased UT receptor levels and found similar results [37]. The mechanism for these changes was later found to be mediated by the activation of the ERK 1/2, p38 and EGFR signalling pathway [28]. Trans-activation of the EGFR results in hypertrophic growth and phenotypic changes in cardiomyocytes that are similar to those observed in heart failure. The activation of hypertrophic growth seen here is induced by a different pathway then that seen in VSMC proliferation, meaning the UTR can act via different pathways to induce proliferative changes following UII binding.UII has also been shown to upregulate procollagen via activation off the TGF-β1 pathway [11, 17], showing further implications in cardiac remodelling and hypertrophy.

RECEPTOR ANTAGONISTS

Given the implications of UII in hypertension, atherosclerosis and heart failure, it is not surprising that UTR antagonists have been proposed as treatment for these pathologies. Although no trials in humans have shown significant results to date, animal trials do show promising results. The UTR antagonist SB-611812 was given to rats following the induction of CHF daily for eight weeks in order to assess any beneficial effects [4]. The treatment group showed reduced ventricular dilation, left ventricular end-diastolic pressure, right ventricular systolic pressure, and central venous pressure when compared to controls. There was also a decrease in pulmonary edema, reduced cardiomyocyte hypertrophy and a reduction in mortality. It was later shown in the same model that the use of SB-611812 was also able to reduce fibrosis and collagen deposition, key factors to cardiac remodelling associated with heart failure [6]. These results suggest that UII is in fact a key player in cardiac dysfunction and blocking its receptor may not only prevent further damage, but potentially reverse the decreased cardiac function seen in CHF patients.

SUMMARY

A better understanding of the pathways involved in the stimulation of the UTR is necessary in order to develop beneficial target drugs. Different pathways are activated by UTR stimulation to cause vasoactive changes, plaque formation, increased foam cells and cardiac hypertrophy, meaning there is a potential for drugs tailored to the pathway mediating negative effects. Using selective inhibitors could be a way to manage an individual component of the disease in a manner which limits side effects. Further studies are needed to investigate the specific conditions involved in UII vasoactivity, particularly the binding of UII to receptors on endothelial cells and VSMC. A better understanding of what receptors and pathways cause vasoactivity could be key to reversing the negative vasoconstriction response initiated by UII in disease states. The varied results of UII vasoactivation could also be explained if UII interacts with other molecules to yield a unique response. This is supported by data suggesting that moxLDL and UII interact to give a synergistic response in atherosclerosis. Discovering these interactions could serve as a means to more easily control the varied effects of UII in diseased tissues.

CONCLUSION

In conclusion, UII has been shown to play a role in the progression of hypertension, the formation of atherosclerotic plaques, increased contraction of the heart and cardiac hypertrophy.

A better understanding of the mechanisms behind these actions is required in order for potential therapeutic drugs to be developed.

ACKNOWLEDGMENT

Dr. Adel Giaid is supported by the Canadian Institute of Health Research and the Quebec Heart Foundation.

REFERENCES

[1]   Ames, RS; Sarau, HM; et al. Human urotensin-II is a potent vasoconstrictor and agonist for the orphan receptor GPR14. *Nature,* 1999, 401, 282-286.

[2]   Bohm, F; Pernow, J. Urotensin II evokes potent vasoconstriction in humans in vivo. *Nature,* 2002, 135, 25-27.

[3]   Bottrill, FE; Douglas, SA; et al. Human urotensin-II is an endothelium-dependent vasodilator in rat small arteries. *Br J Pharmacol,* 2000, 130, 1865-70.

[4]   Bousette, N; Hu, F; et al.: Urotensin-II blockade with SB-611812 attenuates cardiac dysfunction in a rat model of coronary artery ligation. *J Mol Cell Cardiol,* 2006, 41, 285-295.

[5]   Bousette, N; Patel, L; et al. Increased expression of urotensin II and its cognate receptor GPR14 in atherosclerotic lesions of the human aorta. *Atherosclerosis.,* 2004, 176, 117-123.

[6]   Bousette, N; Pottinger, J; et al. Urotensin-II receptor blockade with SB-611812 attenuates cardiac remodeling in experimental ischemic heart disease. *Peptides.,* 2006, 27, 2211-2214.

[7]   Chien, KR; Grace, AA; et al. Molecular Basis of Cardiovascular Disease: biology of cardiac hypertrophy and heart failure. Philadelphia, PA . W.B. Saunders Co., 1998.

[8]   Conlon, JM; Yano, K; et al. Distribution and molecular forms of urotensin-II and its role in cardiovascular regulation in vertebrates. *J Exp Zool,* 1996, 275, 226-38.

[9]   Coulouarn, Y; Jegou, S; et al. Cloning, sequence analysis and tissue distribution of the mouse and rat urotensin II precursors. *FEBS Lett,* 1999, 457, 28-32.

[10]   Coulouarn, Y; Lihrmann, I; et al. Cloning of the cDNA encoding the urotensin II precursor in frog and human reveals intense expression of the urotensin II gene in motoneurons of the spinal cord. *Proc. Natl. Acad. Sci., U. S. A.* 1999, 95, 15803-15808.

[11] Dai, HY; Kang, WQ; et al. The involvement of transforming growth factor-beta1 secretion in urotensin II-induced collagen synthesis in neonatal cardiac fibroblasts. *Regul Pept.*, 2007, 140, 88-93.
[12] Douglas, SA; Tayara, L; et al. Congestive heart failure and expression of myocardial urotensin II. *Lancet*, 2002, 359, 1990-1997
[13] Dschietzig, T; Bartsch, C; et al. Plasma levels and cardiovascular gene expression of urotensin-II in human heart failure. *Regulatory Peptides*, 2002, 110, 33-38.
[14] Grundy, SM. Hypertriglyceridemia, Insulin Resistance, and the Metabolic Syndrome. *Am J Cardiol*, 1999, 83, 25-29.
[15] Gruson, D; Rousseau, MF; et al. Circulating urotensin II levels in moderate to severe congestive heart failure: its relations with myocardial function and well established neurohormonal markers. *Peptides.*, 2006, 27, 1527-1531
[16] Hillier, C; Berry, C; et al. Effects of Urotensin II in Human Arteries and Veins of Varying Caliber. *Circulation*, 2001, 103, 1378-1381.
[17] Kompa, AR; Thomas, WG; et al.: Cardiovascular role of urotensin II: effect of chronic infusion in the rat. *Peptides*, 2004, 25, 1783-1788.
[18] Kruger, S; Graf, J; et al. Urotensin II in patients with chronic heart failure. *The European Journal of Heart Failure*, 2005, 7, 475-478.
[19] Lapp, H; Boerrigter, G; et al. Elevated plasma human urotensin-II-like immunoreactivity in ischemic cardiomyopathy. *International Journal of Cardiology.*, 2004, 94, 93-97.
[20] Levy, D; Garrison, RJ; et al. Prognostic implications of echocardiographically determined left ventricular mass in the Framingham Heart Study. *New England Journal of Medicine.*, 1990, 322, 1561-1566
[21] Levy, D; Larson, M; et al. The progression from hypertension to congestive heart failure. *JAMA.*, 1996, 275, 1557, 1562.
[22] Lim, M; Honisett, S; et al. Differential Effect of Urotensin II on Vascular Tone in Normal Subjects and Patients With Chronic Heart Failure. *Circulation*, 2004, 109, 1212-1215.
[23] MacLean, MR; Alexander, D; et al. Contractile responses to human urotensin-II in rat and human pulmonary arteries: effect of endothelial factors and chronic hypoxia in the rat. *Br. J. Pharmacol, 2000*, 130, 201-204.
[24] Maguire, JJ; Kuc, RE; et al. Cellular distribution of immunoreactive urotensin-II in human tissues with evidence of increased expression in

atherosclerosis and a greater constrictor response of small compared to large coronary arteries. *Peptides.*, 2004, 25, 1767-1774.

[25] Miyazaki, A; Sakashita, N; et al. Expression of ACAT-1 protein in human atherosclerotic lesions and cultured human monocytes-macrophages. *Arterioscler Thromb Vasc Biol.*, 1998, 18, 1568-1574.

[26] Ng, LL; O`Brien, RJ; et al. Plasma Urotensin in Human Systolic Heart Failure. *Circulation.*, 2002, 106, 2877-2880.

[27] Nothacker, HP; Wang, ZAM; et al. Identification of the natural ligand of an orphan G-protein-coupled receptor involved in the regulation of vasoconstriction. *Nat. Cell Biol,* 1999, 1, 383-385.

[28] Onan, D; Pipolo, L; et al. Urotensin II Promotes Hypertrophy of Cardiac Myocytes via Mitogen-Activated Protein Kinase. *Molecular Endocrinology,* 2004, 18, 2344, 2354.

[29] Opgaard, OS; Nothacker, HP; et al. Human urotensin II mediates vasoconstriction via an increase in inositol phosphates. *European Journal of Pharmacology,* 2000, 406, 265-271.

[30] Richards, AM; Nicholls, MG; et al. Plasma urotensin II in heart failure. *Lancet,* 202, 360, 545-546.

[31] Rossowski, WJ; Cheng, BL; et al: Human urotensin II–induced aorta ring contractions are mediated by protein kinase C, tyrosine kinases and Rhokinase: inhibition by somatostatin receptor antagonists. *Eur J Pharmacol,* 2002, 438, 159-170.

[32] Russell, FD; Meyers, D; et al. Elevated plasma levels of human urotensin-II immunoreactivity in congestive heart failure. *AM J Physiol Heart Circ Physiol,* 2003, 285, 1576-1581.

[33] Russell, FD; Molenaar, P. Investigation of signalling pathways that mediate the inotropic effect of urotensin-II in human heart. *Cardiovascular Research.,* 2004, 63, 673-681.

[34] Russell, FD; Molenaar, P; et al. Cardiostimulant effects of urotensin-II in human heart in vitro. *British Journal of Pharmacology.*, 2001, 132, 5-9.

[35] Stirrat, A; Gallagher, M; et al. Potent vasodilator responses to human urotensin-II in humanpulmonary resistance arteries: comparison with adrenomedullin and other vasodilators in pulmonary arteries. *Am J Physiol,* 2001, 280, H925-8.

[36] Tasaki, K; Hori, M; et al. I: Mechanism of human urotensin II–induced contraction in rat aorta. *J Pharmacol Sci,* 2004, 94, 376-383.

[37] Tzanidis, A; Hannan, R; et al. Direct Actions of URotensin II on the Heart. Implications for cardiac fibrosis and hypertrophy. *Circulation Research.*, 2003, 93, 246-253.

[38] Watanabe, T; Kanome, T; et al. Human Urotensin II as a link between hypertension and Coronary Artery Disease. *Hypertension Research,* 2006, 29, 375-387.

[39] Watanabe, T; Pakala, R; et al. Lysophosphatidylcholine and reactive oxygen species mediate the synergistic effect of mildly oxidized LDL with serotonin on vascular smooth muscle cell proliferation. *Circulation.*, 2001, 103, 1440-1445.

[40] Watanabe, T; Pakala, R; et al. Synergistic Effect of Urotensin II With Mildly Oxidized LDL on DNA Synthesis in Vascular Smooth Muscle Cells. *Circulation,* 2001, 104, 16-18.

[41] Watanabe, T; Suguro, T; et al. Human Urotensin II Accelerates Foam Cell Formation in Human Monocyte-Derived Macrophages. *Hypertension,* 2005, 46, 738-744.

[42] Watanabe, T; Takahashi, K; et al. Human Urotensin-II Potentiates the Mitogenic Effect of Mildly Oxidized Low-Density Lipoprotein on Vascular Smooth Muscle Cells: Comparison with Other Vasoactive Agents and Hydrogen Peroxide. *Hypertension Research,* 2006, 29, 821-831.

[43] Wilkinson, IB; Affolter, JT; et al: High plasma concentrations of human urotensin II do not alter local or systemic hemodynamics in man. *Cardiovasc Res,* 2002, 53, 341-347.

[44] Yamazaki, T; Komuro, I; et al. Signalling pathways for cardiac hypertrophy. *Cell. Signal.,* 1998, 10, 693-698.

[45] Zou, Y; Nagai, R; et al. Urotensin II induces hypertrophic responses in cultured cardiomyocytes from neonatal rats. *Federation of European Biochemical Societies Letters.*, 2001, 508, 57-60.

In: Heart Failure: Symptoms, Causes…   ISBN: 978-1-61668-959-9
Editor: Madison S. Wright, pp. 89-101   © 2010 Nova Science Publishers, Inc.

Chapter 5

SHORT COMMUNICATION: IMPACT OF HEALTH-RELATED QUALITY OF LIFE IN OUTPATIENTS WITH HEART FAILURE

Beatriz de Rivas Otero[1], Aida Ribera Solé[2] and Gaietà Permanyer-Miralda[2]

[1] Primary Care Specialist. Madrid. España
[2] Unidad de Epidemiología. Servicio de Cardiología. Hospital Vall d'Hebron.
CIBER de Epidemiología y Salud Pública (CIBERESP), Barcelona.
España

ABSTRACT

Heart failure (HF) is an escalating health problem around the world. Although recent advances in therapy for HF have improved functional capacity and survival, it is becoming increasingly clear that, for many HF patients, improving their quality of life is at least as important as the benefit that a pharmacological treatment may provide with respect to mortality.

Health-related quality of life (HRQL) is a multidimensional concept based on patients own perception of how physical, emotional and social well-being are affected by a disease or its treatment. Studies indicate that HF leads to significant impairment in all aspects of HRQL and that patients with HF have worse HRQL than the general population and patients with other chronic diseases. A worse HRQL in patients with HF has also been associated with hospital readmission and death suggesting that HRQL questionnaires could be a helpful tool to identify patients who are at increased risk of hospital readmission.

However, most published data on HRQL have been obtained from selected, hospital-based patients participating in trials. It is not known how representative they are of patients in the community. Few studies have reported the impact of HF on HRQL in the community, and there is still much less information about the comparison of HRQL in HF patients attended in different health care settings.

Recently, the INCA study evaluated HRQL in unselected outpatients in two different health care levels, Primary Care (PC) and Cardiology outpatient clinics, in Spain. Results of this study have shown that all domains of HRQL were significantly impaired in HF outpatients, and that HRQL (using the EuroQol-5D) was worse in patients with HF than in patients with other chronic diseases such as rheumatoid arthritis or type 2 diabetes, being only comparable to very severe chronic obstructive pulmonary disease. HRQL scores were worse in patients followed in PC than in Cardiology, but differences found could possibly be attributed to a large extent to the different clinical characteristics of the patients attended in each clinical setting. In spite of the differences between EuroQol-5D and Minnesota Living With Heart Failure Questionnaire, the INCA study results suggest that both questionnaires adequately reflect the severity of the disease.

Although the most original feature of the INCA study was the evaluation of HRQL in a presumably representative sample of stable HF attended in two health care settings all over a country, its results agree with the few descriptive data available in outpatients with HF.

These findings emphasize the need for a better knowledge of HRQL in HF in unselected populations, particularly about: 1) The character of its impairment in clinical subgroups; 2) Its association with the patterns of care; 3) Its prognostic meaning and its therapeutic implications; 4) Its implications for public health in the context of chronic diseases.

INTRODUCTION

Heart Failure (HF) is an escalating health problem around the world [1,2]. Patients with HF face significant decreases in functional status, multiple hospital admissions, high mortality, multiple physical and psychological symptoms and a diminished quality of life [3,4]. Although recent advances in therapy for HF have improved functional capacity and survival, it is becoming increasingly clear that, for many HF patients, improving their quality of life is at least as important as the survival benefit that a pharmacological treatment may provide [5]. For this reason, more and more studies are taking quality of life into account and clinical trials have included its measure to evaluate effectiveness of treatment strategies and the course of the disease.

The World Health Organization defines quality of life as "an individual's perception of their position in life in the context of the culture and value systems in which they live and in relation to their goals, expectations, standards and concerns. It is a broad ranging concept affected in a complex way by the person's physical health, psychological state, personal beliefs, social relationships and their relationship to salient features of their environment". In the clinical setting, assessment of quality of life usually concentrates on health-related quality of life (HRQL) which is a multidimensional concept based on patients own perception of how physical, emotional and social well-being are affected by a disease or its treatment [6].

Quality of life outcomes inform us about how patients perceive the disease (subjective information) and the limitations that this perception imposes on them in their daily life. This kind of information cannot be obtained through usual clinical indices, as the New York Heart Association (NYHA) functional class, or objective measures of cardiac function generally used in the clinical setting. Furthermore, HRQL must be self assessed by the patients as it depends on their individual health expectations and perception of functional capacity. So, assessment of HRQL in patients with HF complements traditional measures of clinical effectiveness such as reduction in mortality, hospitalisations and clinical functional measurements.

Measurement of HRQL in Patients with HF

Health-related quality of life instruments may be either generic measures of health status or disease specific. The generic instruments are designed for a wide variety of conditions and offer the possibility to compare HRQL in different diseases and populations. The use of a specific instrument complements the information provided by a generic instrument and provides information on how a disease specifically affects patients' quality of life. Specific instruments are often more sensitive to clinical changes. Although there are several heart failure specific questionnaires such as the Chronic Heart Failure Questionnaire [7], the Yale Scale [8], the Quality of Life Questionnaire in Severe Heart Failure [9], and the Kansas City Cardiomyopathy Questionnaire (KCCQ) [10], the Minnesota Living With Heart Failure

(MWLHF) Questionnaire [11] is the most widely used. The common approach in evaluating HRQL is the combination of a generic and a specific instrument, thus taking advantage of their complementary properties.

Impact of HF in Quality of Life

The impact of HF on patients' quality of life has been evaluated through comparison with samples of the general population and patients with chronic diseases. Studies indicate that heart failure leads to significant impairment in all HRQL dimensions. They also show that patients with HF have worse HRQL than the general population and patients with other chronic diseases such as rheumatoid arthritis, diabetes mellitus, motor neurone disease, Parkinson, hepatitis C, or moderate and severe COPD [6, 12-16]. A similar level of HRQL impairment has been only reported in patients with very severe COPD and chronic haemodialysis [13,15,16].

In general, patients with heart failure have worse scores for health perceptions, physical functioning and role functioning than patients with other chronic conditions [6, 12-16]. As expected, physical condition is better in patients with major depression than in patients with HF. However, patients with HF in NYHA class III have a similar impairment of HRQL in the mental domains as patients with major depression, in addition to their dramatically reduced physical health [13]. These data agree with the finding of some studies showing that a large proportion of patients with HF suffer from depression [17,18]. Thus, HRQL in patients with more severe HF may be reduced not only physically but also mentally.

A recent study [19] has evaluated HRQL in HF patients using the generic questionnaire, the Medical Outcomes Study 36-items Short-Form Survey (SF-36), during hospital admission, after three months and one year after discharge (Figure 1). Results indicate that although all dimensions of HRQL improve, general health perception continues at the same level as discharge. These results are in agreement with the findings of Chin MH et al [20]: SF-36 scores improved at the short term as patients recover from the clinical decompensation and on the whole remained stable or declined slightly over one year.

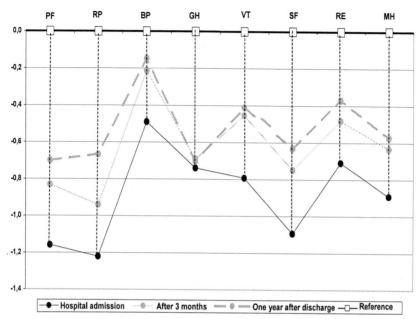

Physical functioning (PF); Role limitations due to physical limitations (RP); Bodily pain (BP); General health perceptions (GH); Vitality (VT); Social functioning (SF); Role limitations caused by emotional problems (RE); Mental health (MH)

Figure 1. Change of mean scores (in number of standard deviations) of the eight components of the Medical Outcomes Study 36-items Short-Form Survey (SF-36) among patients admitted with heart failure relative to the reference Spanish general population scores adjusted by age and sex: during hospital admission, after three months and one year after discharge [19]

Prognostic Value of HRQL

It has been recently demonstrated that the scores obtained on health-related quality of life (HRQL) questionnaires in heart failure patients are related to the severity of the disease [6,13], have prognostic value [21-23] and are also modified by treatment with certain drugs (ACEIs, BBs, ARBs) [24-26]. This fact has aroused interest to evaluate if, in addition to the usual clinical variables, HRQL scores can be used to identify patients who are at special risk for suffering an event (death/hospitalization) and thus are candidates for closer follow-up and more intensive treatment.

The study of Rodríguez-Artalejo F et al [22] was the first to examine the relationship between HRQL and a first emergency rehospitalisation and mortality in a sufficient number of patients with HF and a wide variation in left ventricular ejection fraction (LVEF) and functional status. The study included 394 patients of both sexes who were 65 years and older and were admitted for HF-related emergencies at 4 Spanish hospitals. Baseline HRQL was measured with a generic questionnaire, the SF-36, and with an HF-specific instrument, the MLWHF Questionnaire.

Table 1. Association between HRQL and first emergency rehospitalisation and between HRQL and mortality (adapted of Rodriguez-Artalejo el at) [20]

	Hospital readmission	Death
	Adjusted HR† (95% CI)	Adjusted HR† (95% CI)
SF-36		
Physical functioning	1.65 (1.11-2.44)**	2.08 (1.16-3.72)**
Role-physical	1.26 (0.86-1.86)	1.36 (0.79-2.36)
Bodily pain	1.26 (0.88-1.81)	1.41 (0.82-2.41)
General health	1.73 (1.19-2.52)+	1.72 (1.00-2.96)**
Vitality	1.25 (0.87-1.80)	2.08 (1.22-3.53)+
Social functioning	1.45 (0.99-2.11)	1.71 (0.99-2.95)
Role-emotional	1.38 (0.95-2.00)	1.61 (0.92-2.80)
Mental health	1.65 (1.10-2.47)**	2.46 (1.38-4.40)+
Physical summary score	1.52 (1.04-2.21)**	1.61 (0.93-2.79)
Emotional summary score	1.39 (0.96-2.03)	2.02 (1.15-3.54)**
MLWHF		
Total	1.33 (0.92-1.93)	2.50 (1.42-4.40)+
Physical summary score	1.32 (0.91-1.91)	2.83 (1.60-4.99)*
Emotional summary score	1.41 (0.98-2.04)	1.93 (1.12-3.33)**

Abbreviation: CI, confidence interval; HR, hazard ratio; HRQL, health-related quality of life; SF-36, Medical Outcomes Study 36-Items Short-Form Survey; MLWHF, Minnesota Living With Heart Failure questionnaire

† Adjusted for age; sex; educational level; personal history of myocardial infarction, diabetes mellitus, and chronic pulmonary disease; cause of heart failure; left ventricular ejection fraction; functional grade (New York Heart Association classification); Charlson Index; plasma creatinine level; plasma sodium level; instability at hospital discharge; treatment at discharge with angiotensin-converting enzyme inhibitor, β-blocker, and digitalis; a physician opinion of poor treatment compliance; previous hospitalization for heart failure in the past year; duration of stay at index hospitalization; influenza vaccination; and hospital center.

* P <0.001 ** P <0.05 + P <0.01

During a median follow up of about 6 months, 35% of patients underwent a first emergency rehospitalisation and 17.8% died. After adjustment for biomedical, psychosocial, and health care variables, the frequency of death was higher in patients with worse scores on the SF-36 physical functioning (HR, 2.08; 95% confidence interval [CI], 1.16-3.72; P<0.05), general health (HR, 1.72; 95% CI, 1.00-2.96; P<0.05), and mental health (HR, 2.46; 95% CI, 1.38-4.40; P<0.01) subscales. Results were similar for the hospital readmission end point. For the MLWHF questionnaire, worse overall and worse physical and emotional summary scores were associated with higher mortality (Table 1).

Thus, worse HRQL was associated with hospital readmission and death in patients with HF. The magnitude of this association, for both physical and mental HRQL components, was comparable to that for other well-known predictors of hospital readmission and death, such as personal history of diabetes, previous hospitalizations, and treatment with angiotensin-converting enzyme inhibitors. The results of this study showed that short, simple HRQL questionnaires could be useful to identify patients who are at a relatively higher risk of hospital readmission and death. Such patients could benefit from closer follow-up, and their eligibility for inclusion in disease management programs should be assessed.

HRQL in Outpatients

Most published data on HRQL in patients with heart failure have been obtained from selected, hospital-based patients participating in trials. It is not known how representative they are of patients in the community. Few studies have reported the impact of HF on HRQL in the community and there is still much less information about the comparison of HRQL in HF patients attended in different health care settings.

Recently, the INCA study evaluated the global impact of heart failure in an unselected large number of outpatients in Spain, and compared the HRQL perceptions between patients follow-up in Primary Care and in Cardiology outpatients clinics all over Spain [15].

This cross-sectional study included 2161 (1412 in Primary Care; 749 in Cardiology) stable patients diagnosed of chronic heart failure on a clinical and echocardiographic basis. HRQL was evaluated with a generic questionnaire: the EuroQol 5D (EQ-5D) and a disease-specific instrument: the Minnesota Living with Heart Failure Questionnaire (MLWHF).

Patients followed up in Cardiology were younger (mean age in Cardiology 68.5 *vs* 72.2 years in Primary Care; p<0.0001), and with greater male predominance (63.32% in Cardiology *vs* 51.58% in Primary Care; P <0.0001). They had better functional class (NYHA in Cardiology: I 15.92%, II 60.54%, III 22.45%, IV 1.09% *vs* NYHA in Primary Care: I 16.05%, II 49.48%, III 30.92%, IV 3.55%; P <0.0001), lower ejection fraction (EF) (mean EF in Cardiology 44.2 *vs* 49.5 in Primary Care; P <0.0001), and fewer co-morbidities (88.79% in Cardiology *vs* 96.74%; P <0.0001) than those followed in Primary Care.

The results of the INCA study showed that chronic heart failure significantly affects all dimensions of quality of life in patients with stable disease who are attended either in Primary Care or in Cardiology. HRQL scores were worse in patients followed in Primary Care than in patients followed in Cardiology (Table 2). After adjusting for clinical variables (functional class, gender, age and non cardiovascular co-morbidity) the differences between Primary Care and Cardiology disappeared in the summary (mean score 45.1 in Cardiology *vs* 44.9 in Primary Care; P =0.87) and physical MLWHF score (mean score 20.0 in Cardiology *vs* 20.1 in Primary Care; P =0.80), but persisted to a smaller degree in EQ-5D index (mean index 0.57 in Cardiology *vs* 0.54 in Primary Care; P <0.05), EQ-VAS (mean score 55.1 in Cardiology *vs* 52.5 in Primary Care; P <0.05) and mental MLWHF (mean score 10.2 in Cardiology *vs* 10.8 in Primary Care; P =0.03).

The differences in the clinical characteristics of the patients attended in one setting or the other probably determined to a large extent the differences in quality of life observed. Nevertheless, the fact that the differences disappeared to a greater extent on the specific than on the generic questionnaire may suggest that the generic questionnaire captures general health perceptions better than the specific questionnaire, which focuses on the functional limitations specific to the disease. The fact that after adjustment a small difference persists in precisely the emotional dimension of MLWHF questionnaire is also compatible with this interpretation.

In order to assess the impact of HF on HRQL, the INCA study compared the mean visual analogue self-rating scale (EQ VAS) score of the EQ-5D questionnaire with a representative sample of Spanish population and with the results from available studies with other chronic conditions. Results indicated that HRQL was worse in INCA than in a representative sample of the Spanish population, and was also apparently worse than in other chronic conditions such as rheumatoid arthritis or type 2 diabetes, being only comparable to very severe COPD (Table 3).

The INCA study in out-patients with HF [15] and the CARE-HF study in HF patients with left ventricular systolic dysfunction included in a clinical trial [6] evaluated HRQL using simultaneously a generic (the EQ-5D) and a disease-specific questionnaire (the MLWHF questionnaire). In both studies, a statistically significant correlation was found between the score obtained on the EQ-5D and the MLWHF. Both questionnaires also showed that they adequately reflected the severity of the disease.

Table 2. Results of the HRQL questionnaires, comparing Primary Care and Cardiology outpatients clinics (Adapted from De Rivas B et al) [15]

	Primary Care	Cardiology	p
EQ-5D descriptive [% patients with any problem, (CI 95%)] Mobility Self-care Usual activities Pain/discomfort Anxiety/depression	66 (63.4,68.4) 37 (34.4,39.5) 65.2 (62.7,67.7) 64.6 (62.1,67.1) 55.2 (52.6,57.9)	62.7 (59.3,66.2) 28.6 (25.4,31.9) 53.8 (50.3,57.4) 50.1 (46.5,53.7) 44.9 (41.3,48.5)	0.18 <0.05 <0.05 <0.05 <0.05
Mean EQ-5D index, (CI 95%) (min HRQL -0.594 - max 1)	0.60 (0.59,0.61)	0.68 (0.66,0.69)	<0.05
Mean EQ-VAS score, (CI 95%) (min HRQL 0 - max 100)	55.8 (54.9,56.7)	61.0 (59.8,62.2)	<0.05
Mean summary MLWHF score (min HRQL 105 - max 0), (IC 95%) -Physical score (min 40- max 0) -Mental score (min 25- max 0)	40.8 (39.8,41.9) 18.4 (17.9,18.8) 9.8 (9.5,10.1)	38.1 (36.7,39.6) 16.8 (16.2,17.5) 8.4 (8.0,8.8)	<0.05 <0.05 <0.05

Abbreviation: HRQL, health-related quality of life; EQ-5D, EuroQol 5D; CI, confidence interval; EQ-VAS, EuroQol visual analogue scale; MLWHF, Minnesota Living With Heart Failure questionnaire

Table 3. Comparison of EQ-VAS INCA results with normal population and other chronic diseases other than HF (Adapted from De Rivas B et al) [15]

	EQ-VAS (mean ± SD)	p vs INCA
INCA	57.6±16.7	
Spanish population	71.1±18	<0.05
Rheumatoid arthritis	65.0±19.3	<0.05
COPD		
Moderate	67.7±15.7	<0.05
Severe	62.4±17.0	<0.05
Very severe	57.8±16.2	0.91
Diabetes Mellitus	61.7±18.6	<0.05

Abbreviation: EQ-VAS, EuroQol visual analogue scale; HF, heart failure; COPD, chronic obstructive pulmonary disease

The high response rate obtained on the EQ-5D in these and other studies, along with the simplicity and rapidity of its administration and the demonstration of its relationship with the score on the MLWHF questionnaire and the severity of heart failure, suggest that the EQ-5D may be a valid and acceptable way to measure quality of life of patients with heart failure. This observation could be particularly useful for clinical purposes when the attending physicians, especially in Primary Care, have little time available for each patient. However, further studies are needed to evaluate the prognostic value of this questionnaire and its true clinical utility in the evaluation and follow-up of these patients.

CONCLUSIONS

All these data indicate that all domains of HRQL are significantly impaired in HF patients. HRQL is worse in these patients than in the general population and in other chronic conditions. And this is true both for hospital-based patients with HF participating in trials and for outpatients with HF.

Scores obtained on HRQL questionnaires in HF patients are also related to the severity of the disease [6,13], have prognostic value [21-23], and in addition to the usual clinical variables, could be used to identify patients who are at special risk for suffering an event (death/hospitalization) and thus are candidates for closer follow-up and more intensive treatment. So, systematically registering HRQL in clinical practice during the follow up of patients with HF would be useful to increase the collective experience. These data might give information about the evolution of scores with time and the prognostic meaning that such evolution could have.

In spite of the differences between a generic and a HF-specific questionnaire, such as EQ-5D and MLWHF, results from studies suggest that both questionnaires adequately reflect the severity of the disease. So, the choice of the instrument to measure HRQL in clinical practice depends on what we are looking for (a global measure of global health or concrete aspects) and on the time available to evaluate HRQL in each patient. In this sense the EQ-5D, due to its simplicity of administration, could be useful to evaluate quality of life of patients with HF. However, for research purposes wider instruments or the combination of generic and specific questionnaire appears as more promising

These findings also emphasize the need for a better knowledge of HRQL in HF in unselected populations, particularly about: 1) The character of its impairment in clinical subgroups; 2) Its association with the patterns of care; 3) Its prognostic meaning and its therapeutic implications; 4) Its implications for public health in the context of chronic diseases.

REFERENCES

[1]   Stewart, S; MacIntyre, K; Capewell, S; et al. Heart failure and the aging population: an increasing burden in the 21st century?. *Heart*, 2003, 89, 49-53.

[2]   Young, JB. The global epidemiology of heart failure. *Med Clin North Am*, 2004, 88, 1135-43.

[3]   Rodriguez-Artalejo, F; Banegas Banegas, JR; Guallar-Castillón, P. Epidemiology of heart failure. *Rev Esp Cardiolo*, 2004, 57, 163-70.

[4]   Archana, R; Gray, D. The quality of life in chronic-disease-heart failure is as bad as it gets. *Eur Heart J*, 2002, 23, 1806-8.

[5]   Lewis, EF; Johnson, PA; Johnson, W; et al. Preferences for quality of life or survival expressed by patients with heart failure. *J Heart Lung Transplant*, 2001, 20, 1016-24.

[6]   Calvert, MJ; Freemantle, N; Cleland, JGF. The impact of chronic heart failure on health-related quality of life data acquired in the baseline phase of the CARE-HF study. *Eur J Heart Fail*, 2005, 7, 243-51.

[7]   Guyatt, GH; Nogradi, S; Halcrow, S. Development and testing of a new measure of health status for clinical trials in heart failure. *J Gen Intern Med*, 1989, 4, 101-7.

[8]   Feinstein, AR; Fisher, MB; Pigeon, JG. Changes in dyspnea-fatigue ratings as indicators of quality of life in the treatment of congestive heart failure. *Am J Cardiol*, 1989, 64, 50-5

[9]   Wiklund, I; Lindvall, K; Swedberg, K; et al. Self-assessment of quality if life in severe heart failure. *Scand J Psychol*, 1987, 28, 220-5.

[10]   Green, CP; Porter, CB; Bresnahan, DR; et al. Development and evaluation of the Kansas City Cardiomyopathy Questionnaire: a new status measure for heart failure. *JACC*, 2000, 35, 1245-55.

[11]   Rector, TS; Kubo, SH; Cohn, JN. Patients' self-assessment of their congestive heart failure, part 2: content, reliability and validity of a new measure, the Minnesota Living With Heart Failure Questionnaire. *Heart Fail*, 1987, 3, 198-209.

[12]   Stewart, AL; Greenfield, S; Hays, RD; et al. Functional status and well-being of patients with chronic conditions. Results from the Medical Outcomes Study. Journal of the *American Medical Association*, 1989, 262, 907-13.

[13]   Juenger, J; Schellberg, D; Kraemer, S; et al. Health related quality of life in patients with congestive heart failure: comparison with other chronic diseases and relation to functional variables. *Heart*, 2002, 87, 235-41.

[14]   Hobbs, FD; Kenkre, JE; Roalfe, AK; et al. Impact of heart failure and left ventricular systolic dysfunction on quality of life. *Eur Heart J*, 2002, 23, 1867-76

[15]   De Rivas, B; Permanyer-Miralda, G; Brotons C et al. Health-reated quality of life in unselected outpatients with heart failure across Spain in two different health care levels. Magnitude and determinants of impairment: The INCA study. *Qual of Life Res*, 2008, 17, 1229-1238

[16]   Merkus, MP; Jager, KJ; Dekker, FW; et al. Quality of life in patients on chronic dialysis *Am J Kidney Dis*, 1997, 29, 584-92.

[17]   Murberg, TA; Bru, E; Svebak, S; et al. Depressed mood and subjective health symptoms as predictors of mortality in patients with congestive heart failure. *Int J Psychiatry Med*, 1999, 29, 311-26.

[18]   Havranek, EP; Ware, MG; Lowes, BD. Prevalence of depression in congestive heart failure. *Am J Cardiol*, 1999, 84, 348-50.

[19] Soriano, N; Permanyer-Miralda, G; Ribera, A; et al. Health related quality of life evolution in a population of patients with heart failure. IC-QoL study. Rev Esp Cardiol 2010 (in press)

[20] Chin, MH; Goldman, L. Gender differences in 1-year survival and quality of life among patients admitted with congestive heart failure. *Med Care*, 1998, 36, 1033-46

[21] Alla, F; Briancon, S; Guillemin, F; et al. Selfrating of quality of life provides additional prognostic information in heart failure. Insights into the EPICAL study. *Eur J Heart* Fail, 2002, 4, 337-43

[22] Rodriguez-Artalejo, F; Guallar-Castillón, P; Rodríguez Pascual, C; et al. Health-related quality of liffe as a predictor of hospital readmision and death among patients with heart failure. *Arch Intern Med*, 2005, 165, 1274-79.

[23] Konstam, V; Salem, D; Pouleur, H; et al. Baseline quality of life as a predictor of mortality and hospitalisation in 5,025 patients with congestive heart failure. *Am J Cardiol*, 1996, 78, 890-5.

[24] Rector, TD; Kubo, SH; Cohn, JN. Validity of the Minnesota Living With Heart Failure Questionnaire as a measure of therapeutic response to enalapril. *Am J Cardiol*, 1993, 71, 1106-7.

[25] Rogers, WJ; Johnstone, DE; Yusuf, S; et al. Quality of life among 5,025 patients with left ventricular dysfunction randomised between placebo and enalapril: the studies of left ventricular dysfunction. The SOLVD investigators. *J Am Coll Cardiol*, 1994, 23, 393-400.

[26] Majani, G; Giardini, A; Opasichi, C; et al. Effect of valsartan on quality of life when added to usual therapy for heart failure: results from the valsartan heart failure trial. *J Card Fail*, 2005, 11, 253-9.

In: Heart Failure: Symptoms, Causes...   ISBN: 978-1-61668-959-9
Editor: Madison S. Wright, pp. 103-110 © 2010 Nova Science Publishers, Inc.

Chapter 6

PERSPECTIVE DIRECTION IN BIOMEDICAL NANOTECHNOLOGIES FOR HEART FAILURE DIAGNOSTICS AND TREATMENT

Sergei Yu. Zaitsev*

Department of Organic and Biological Chemistry, FGOY VPO "Moscow State
Academy of Veterinary Medicine and Biotechnology named after K. I.
Skryabin", Moscow, Russia

ABSTRACT

The advanced research in the field of biomedical nanotechnologies is concentrating on the following directions: fundamental studies of principles for the formation and function of biological nanodimensional systems; application of the acquired knowledge to the design of novel bionanomaterials, bionanotechnological processes and bio-nanodimensional devices; as well as particular technologies for local selective diagnostics, therapy, surgery, gene engineering and biotechnology. The enormous activity in these fields is connected with the recent achievements in cell biochemistry and molecular biology, as well as with the development of powerful physical-chemical methods and equipment. Our research is concentrating on the design of nanomaterials

* Corresponding author: FAX: 495-3774939, szaitsev@mail.ru

for the sensing system of a biomedical robot. This robot will operate in the blood vessels (such as arteries and veins) for local selective diagnostics and treatment of venous and arterial thrombosis.

Biomedical Nanotechnology (biomednanotehnology) is an important new field on the "so-called crossroads" of biomedical, biochemical, veterinary, physical-technical and some other sciences, studying the principles of creation and function of biological nanostructures; application of acquired knowledge for improving existing and developing innovative bionanomaterials, biotechnological processes and "bionanosized" devices; new nanotechnologies for local selective diagnostics, therapy, surgery, genetic engineering and biotechnology. Active development of this area is associated with major advances in biochemistry and molecular biology of cell, in modeling and understanding the molecular mechanisms of cellular and subcellular system structure and functions, and with development of new methods for the study of nanoscale biosystems, physiological-biochemical parameters in organism of animals and humans [1]. Even some complex proteins (chromoproteins, metaloproteins, lipoproteins, glycoproteins, etc.) and enzyme-substrate (Figure 1) complexes can be regarded as natural nanodimensional systems, structurally and functionally optimized during evolution (Figure 1). Moreover, it relates to their supramolecular systems such as biological membranes (Figure 2), formed by the fundamental principles of self-association and molecular recognition [2-4].

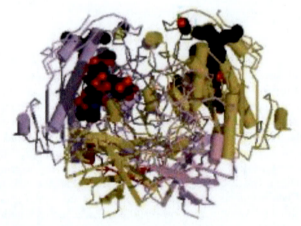

Figure 1 Continued

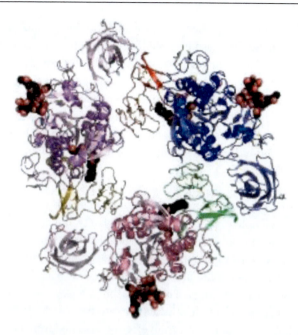

Figure 1. Schematic representation of supramolecular systems of molecules of the substrate and the dimer (left) and oktamera (right) complexes of pancreatic lipase from pig (Sus scrofa): [code 1eth from PDB-EBI]

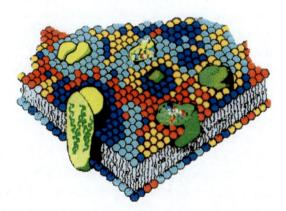

Figure 2. Schematic presentation of the biological membrane [11]

In recent years, several books and reviews of Russian scientists on various aspects of nanotechnology and bionanotechnology [5-11], reflecting the approaches to the creation of supramolecular biosystems and protein complexes with desired properties through self-association of macromolecules, electronic nanodevices (based on metalloproteins), photochromic and photorefractive materials (based on photosensitive proteins nanoelements) for optical memory and thin-film displays (based on bacteriorhodopsin), processes of controlled self-assembly of proteins, functional protein complexes for biotechnological processes, therapeutic nanodevices, etc. The actual application on a global scale of various developed bionanomaterials, biotechnological processes and bionanosize devices in all sectors of the economy, including biology, medicine and veterinary medicine, is expected in the nearest 10-15 years [6-11].

In fact, some laboratory developments in these areas already exist, but their implementation requires a large-scale development procedures as well as convincing and complete set of data on their safety for humans and animals. Among the main biomednanotechnology developments one should mention the "nano-carriers" for targeted delivery of drugs, which will "overcome" the problem of poor solubility and absorption of new drugs, as well as to radically reduce the doses of toxic drugs. This approach is based on the use of natural biopolymer particles of nucleic acids or proteins and synthetic polymer particles on special copolymers, polyelectrolytes, dendrimers, etc. In such particle cavity it is possible to incorporate various biologically active substances (BAS) that becomes chemically inert and less toxic to the organism. Such compounds are promising for X-ray diagnosis (as many modern compounds more toxic and rapidly disintegrate in the body); for creation of some drug compositions (which release the active substance only when it reach the target cell); for creation of the novel antioxidants and antiallergenic substances. On the other hand, different types of nanoparticles (lipid, polypeptide, polymer, etc.) ranging in size from 10 to 100 nm are suggested for immobilization of various BAS at their surface with further application in drug delivery systems designed to organs and tissues of humans and animals.

The most amazing achievements in the field of biomednanotehnology are "so-called" micro- and nanodimensional "robots" capable of "repairing" damaged cells and tissues, diagnosis and treatment of oncological diseases, mapped and cleared of cholesterol blood vessels. The increasing activity in these modern areas are currently observed in some international and Russian research groups (one of those in the Department of Organic and Biological Chemistry of MSAVM&B is currently working under author's leadership) [11-17]. The aim of the project is to create "mikrorobototechnical complex on the basis of intravascular robot for the implementation of diagnostic, therapeutic (drug targeting) and surgical procedures for atherosclerotic disease

of the tubular bodies" [17] (Figure 3). We performed a section associated with the creation of diagnostic systems and methods for the determination of cations and small organic molecules in model and biological liquids [12-16]. Together with scientists Photochemistry Center of the Russian Academy of Sciences (leading by prof. S. P. Gromov) we developed techniques and obtained a series of samples of nanocomposite materials (NCM) on the basis of new membrane-active compounds (MAC), for detection of various cations and BAS in the biological and model liquids that described in a number of joint publications [12-16]. There are three of the fluorescence spectrum NCM (containing the MAC in a polymer matrix) in the presence of diamines such propandiammony perchlorate (PDA) in low concentrations (0.1-1.0 mM) causes significant shifts of maximum fluorescence (on 23-31 nm, respectively) and intensity (Figure 4.). These changes are sufficient for design of the optical detection system of intravascular "robot" connected by the transmission fiber to the control center (with computer) located outside of the human's or animal's organism. These data make the requested NCM (based on polymer composition MAS) the most promising for PDA detection as a model compound for a variety of N-containing BAS.

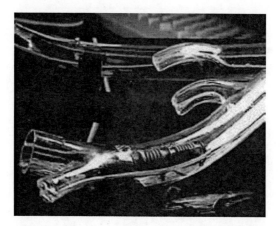

Figure 3. Scheme of the "biorobot in the vessel": developed in the frame of the integrated project on the topic "Creating bitmap detection system of intravascular microrobot for collecting information about the situation inside the bioobject cavity " for 2007-2009 years between by MSTU named N.E. Bauman, the Center of Photochemistry RAS, the Department of Organic and Biological Chemistry MSAVM&B on the state contract "Creating microrobotechnical complex on the basis of intravascular microrobot for diagnostic, therapeutic (drug targeting) and surgical procedures for atherosclerotic disease of the tubular organs" by Russian Ministry of Education and Science [17]

It is important to underline that a reliable biomedical robot can be more precisely defined as "mircometer-sized device (based on nanodimensional complex elements and systems) operating in the blood vessels" [17] than as "nanodevice that can enter cells and organells to interact directly with DNA and proteins" [18].

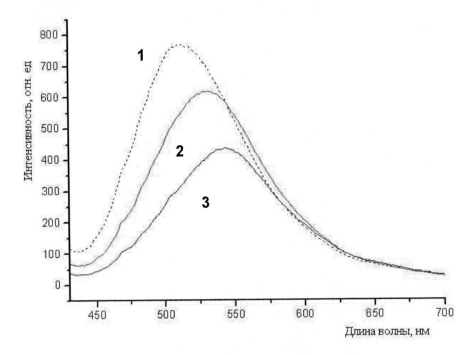

Figure 4. Fluorescence spectra of nanocomposite materials (NCM) before (curve 1, dotted line) and after (curves 2, 3) treatment with a solution propandiaamina PDA with a concentration of 0.1 mM (curve 2, red) or 1.0 mM (curve 3, blue)

These results are only one example of numerous data obtained as a result of our work over the past years [12-16], showing great potential of the biomedical nanotechnology.

REFERENCES

[1] Zaitsev, S. (2009). Yu. *Russian nanotehnology, v.4,* №.7-8., 6-18.
[2] Ahlers, M., Mueller, W., Reichert, A., Ringsdorf, H. & Venzmer, J. (1990). Angew. Chem., Int. *Ed. Engl., v.29,* 1269-1285.

[3] Gennis, G. (1997). Biomembranes: molecular structure and function, M. *Mir*, 624.

[4] Zaitsev, S. (1998). Yu. Rossijskij himicheskij zhurnal. Journal RHO named D. I. *Mendeleev.*, *v.42*, №1-2, 103-115 (in Russain).

[5] Alfimov, M. V. & Razumov, V. F. (2007). *Russian nanotehnology.*, *v.2*, №1-2, 12-25.

[6] Gromov, S. P. (2006). *Russian nanotehnology.*, *v.1*, №1-2, 29-45.

[7] Kiselev, G. A. & Jaminskij, I. V. (2007). *Russian nanotehnology.*, *v.2*, №9-10, 112-117.

[8] Kulichihin, V. G., Antonov, S. V., Makarova, V. V., Semakov, A. V. & Singh, R. (2006). *Russian nanotehnology.*, *v.1*, №1-2, 170-181.

[9] Glazko, V. I. & Belopuhov, S. L. (2008). Nanotehnologii v sel'skom hozjajstve. Moscow: RGAU-MSHA imeni K.A. *Timirjazeva*, *112*, (in Russain).

[10] Bovin, N. V., Tuzikov, A. B., Chinarev, A. A. & Gambarjan, A. S. (2004). *Molekuljarnaja medicina.*, *3*, 56-61 (in Russain).

[11] Zaitsev, S. (2006). Yu. Supramolekuljarnye sistemy na granice razdela faz kak modeli biomembran i nanomaterialy. Doneck, Moscow: *Nord Komp'juter.*, *189*, (in Russain).

[12] Zaitsev S. Yu., Bondarenko, V. V., Varlamova, E. A., Staroverova, I. N., Frolova, L. A. & Tsarkova, M. S. (2006). Uchenye zapiski Kazanskoj gosudarstvennoj akademii veterinarnoj *mediciny.*, *v.186*, 141-148 (in Russain).

[13] Bondarenko, V. V., Zaitsev, S. Yu., Tsarkova, M. S., Varlamova, E. A., Kordonskaja, M. A., Staroverova, I. N., Dmitrieva, S. N., Gromov, S. P. & Alfimov, M. V. (2007). Izvestija VUZov. *Chemistry & Chem. tehnology.*, v.50, №11, 25-28 (in Russain).

[14] Zaitsev, S. Yu., Varlamova, E. A., Tsarkova, M. S., Staroverova, I. N., Gogasov, K. A., Gromov, S. P., Alfimov, M. V., Turshatov, A. A. & Moebius, D. (2006). *Mendeleev Communications.*, *v. 16*, №6, 300-301.

[15] Zaitsev, S. Yu., Zarudnaya, E. N., Moebius, D., Bondarenko, V. V., Maksimov, V. I., Gromov, S. P. & Alfimov, M. V. (2008). *Mendeleev Communications. v. 18*, №6, 270-272.

[16] Zaitsev, S. Yu., Tsarkova, M. S., Varlamova, E. A., Bondarenko, V. V., Timonin, A. N., Lobova, N. A., Vedernikov, A. I., Gromov, S. P., Alfimov, M. V. Izvestija, VUZov. *Chemistry & Chem. tehnology.* 2009, V.52, 65-69 (in Russain).

[17] Zaitsev, S. Yu. (2009). Supramolecular nanodimensional systems at interfaces : concepts and perspectives for bionanotechnology. M: URSS, 208, (in Russain).

[18] Tachung, C. (2005). Yih, Chiming Wei. *Nanomedicine, v.1*, 191-192.

In: Heart Failure: Symptoms, Causes...   ISBN: 978-1-61668-959-9
Editor: Madison S. Wright, pp. 111-114 © 2010 Nova Science Publishers, Inc.

Chapter 7

COMMENTARY

Nan Li

Division of Clinical Pharmacology and Cardiology, Sir Run Run Shaw
Hospital,
School of Medicine, Zhejiang University, Hangzhou, China

Heart failure is a major and growing public health problem in the United States as well as in the whole world. With increasing morbidity and mortality, it is primarily developed in the elderly population. The cost for the diagnosis and treatment of heart failure cause a heavy burden to the whole society.

It is crucial for a medical professional to critically evaluate diagnostic methods and therapies during the detection, management and prevention of heart failure. Heart failure is a progressive cardiac disorder. Diagnosis and appropriate treatment of heart failure at Stage A and stage B can prevent the advance to the next Stage C and Stage D. It is recognized that at stage C or Stage D, even NYHA functional class varies in response to therapy or to the progression of disease, it is impossible for a patient to reverse to Stage B. Emphasis on prevention of heart failure from stage A & B to Stage C & D is therefore utmost important.

With reference to 2009 ACC/AHA heart failure guideline in 2009, state of the art diagnostic approaches are medical history, physical examination and serum natriuretic peptides level determination. Currently BNP is recommended by 2009 ACC/AHA heart failure guideline to be in the context of overall evaluation of heart failure. Measurement of BNP or NT-BNP can be helpful in differential diagnosis when heart failure is uncertain.   For example, a level of BNP over 400 pg/ml is helpful to diagnose heart failure from other diseases.   However, is it meaningful for a minor or moderate elevation of BNP level such as from 5 pg/ml to 400 pg/ml?   Is BNP in isolation or with other lab biomarkers helpful to predict high risks of heart failure as indicated in the below? Its potential role in early prediction of heart failure with high risks warrants numerous studies.

BNP alone or with other lab biomarkers

Hypertension and hypertrophy
Coronary artery disease and angina
AMI
Old AMI and LV hypertrophy

Prevention of remodeling is an expected therapeutic target of heart failure treatment. It is unclear yet whether remodeling can be reversed to a previous stage or not. At least the benefit of such therapy is to prevent advance of remodeling to next stage.

Besides taking morbidity and mortality as hard markers, many surrogate markers of remodeling can be practically used to reflect maladaptive remodeling situation at myocyte level. The myocyte stands in the center of remodeling process, accompanying with interstitium and vasculature. These changes include re-expression of fatal gene program, alteration of sarcolemma, sarcoplastic reticulum, and mitochondria, alteration of energy metabolism, alteration of excitation-contraction of coupling, alteration of myofibrillar and content and function, alteration of nutrient homeostasis, myocyte hypertrophy, myocyte apoptosis, and myocyte necrosis. Changes in vasculature include endocellular dysfunction, intima thickening, smooth muscle hyperplasia, and rarefaction of capillary. Alteration of interstitium is found in increased collagen synthesis and fibrosis, myocyte slipping, collagen isoform shift, and matrix metalloproteases induction. The relevant process of ischemia, apoptosis and necrosis are presented. As results, progressive reduction of systolic and diastolic function, development of mitral regurgitation, and increase of arrhythmias are found.

Normal energy metabolism in heart failure is impaired.   Fatty acid oxidation is shifted to less oxygen required glucose derived energy production.

Positive   reverse   remodeling   approaches   are   evident   in   non pharmacological therapies such as long term moderate exercise training and continuous positive airway pressure therapy. Evident reverse remodeling pharmacological therapies are ACEI, aldosterone receptor blockage, and beta-blockers.

Novel pharmacological therapy includes nesiritide, testosterone, and so on. While evident surgical therapies are cardiac resynchronization therapy, ventricular restoration surgery. MicroRNA may play an important role in the regulation of the gene expression that governs the adaptive and maladaptive medical device, gene therapy and stem cell transplantation are under investigation.

According to the guideline evidence-based treatment of heart failure includes: general therapies, routine drug therapies (ACEI and beta-blockers) and selective interventions. There are many interventions are under investigation such as dietary intervention, exercise training, novel drug interventions, medical device approaches, surgical approaches such as surgical ventricular restoration, gene therapy and stem cell transplantation.

In detail, various clinical trials are investigated using following approaches:

omega-3 polyunsaturated fatty acid
correction of anemia
inspiratory muscle training
BNP
Statins
Biventricular pacing
Surgical ventricular restoration
Autologous meshenchymal stem cell transplantation

The most promising dietary intervention is fish n-3 polyunsaturated fatty acid. In laboratory studies, n-3 PUFA has a direct modulation of gene profile on cardiomyocytes. Its recognized cardioprotective effects are evident by randomized, double blind, placebo-controlled clinical trial such as GISSI-HF trial.

Further, numerous translational preclinical studies are as follows:

microRNA
PARP inhibition
TNF-alpha inhibition
Modulation of nitric oxide pathways
Inhibition of inflammation and proteolysis
Inhibition of protein tyrosine phosphatase 1B

Inhibition of mitochondria oxidant stress

Angiogenesis

Heart failure is also increasingly recognized as a multisystem disorder characterized as anemia, cardiac cachexia, increased systolic tone, hormone derangement, metabolism unbalance, endothelia dysfunction, and systemic low-grade inflammation. Gut is playing a pathophysiological role in the chronic inflammation and malnutrition. There are alterations in intestinal morphology, permeability and absorption function.

Dietary intervention shall be highlighted as simple and cheap approaches may effectively correct anemia, provide abundant n-3 PUFA and extenuate system inflammation. Long moderate exercise shall be emphasized as it may improve HF patients' quality of life, survival and remodeling. The most cost-effective strategy is to prevent the advance of stage A & B to next stage, which is real heart failure.

In: Heart Failure: Symptoms, Causes...   ISBN: 978-1-61668-959-9
Editor: Madison S. Wright, pp. 115-141 © 2010 Nova Science Publishers, Inc.

Chapter 8

SUDDEN CARDIAC DEATH RISK STRATIFICATION IN HEART FAILURE –THE POTENTIAL ROLE OF BIOMARKERS

P. A. Scott[1], J. M. Morgan[1] and P. A. Townsend[2]*
[1]Wessex Cardiothoracic Centre, Southampton University Hospitals NHS Trust,
SO16 6YD, UK
[2] Human Genetics Division, University of Southampton, SO16 6YD,UK

ABSTRACT

Although there has been significant recent progress in the management of heart failure its associated mortality remains high. A large proportion of these patients die suddenly, termed sudden cardiac death (SCD), mostly from potentially reversible malignant cardiac arrhythmias. Despite the availability of a highly effective treatment in the form of an implantable cardioverter defibrillator (ICD), SCD in the heart

---

* Corresponding author: Reader in Molecular Cell Biology and Head of Transcription Regulation Group Human Genetics Division, Duthie Building MP808, Southampton General Hospital, Tremona Road, Southampton, SO16 6YD, UK, 023 80 798692 (tel), 023 89 794264 (fax), p.a.townsend@soton.ac.uk

failure population is still a significant problem. One important reason for this is the difficulty in identifying which patients are at highest risk of SCD and would benefit from an ICD. A number of tests are currently available to risk stratify heart failure patients at risk of SCD. However, used alone or in combination these are not sufficiently accurate and there is significant need for better risk stratification tools.

Multiple studies have demonstrated that serum biomarkers can accurately predict adverse outcomes in patients with heart failure of both ischaemic and non-ischaemic aetiology. A range of biomarkers predict both the occurrence of SCD in patients without ICDs and the occurrence of malignant arrhythmias in patients with devices, and in these studies individual biomarkers are at least as accurate as the current best markers of SCD risk. The pathophysiology of SCD is a complex process with a range of electro-physiological and molecular alterations contributing to arrhythmogenesis in the failing heart. By providing an assessment of these various processes, serum biomarkers may improve prediction of SCD in heart failure and help guide ICD use. Furthermore, it is likely that optimal SCD risk stratification will require the combination of multiple tests that reflect these diverse upstream processes. As such the greatest potential benefit of biomarkers may be in measuring multiple complementary markers that assess distinct aspects of arrhythmic risk.

INTRODUCTION

There has been significant recent progress in the management of heart failure with advances in neurohormonal blockade and the advent of device therapy. In spite of this the mortality associated with heart failure remains high - 80% of men and 70% of women under the age 65 with heart failure will die within 8 years [1]. A large proportion of these patients die suddenly, termed sudden cardiac death (SCD), mostly from potentially reversible malignant arrhythmias. Despite the availability of a highly effective treatment, in the form of an implantable cardioverter defibrillator (ICD), SCD in the heart failure population is still a significant problem. One important reason for this is the difficulty in identifying which patients are at highest risk of SCD and would benefit from an ICD. In this chapter we review the importance and pathophysiology of SCD in heart failure, detail the currently available tools for SCD risk stratification, and consider the potential role of biomarkers.

THE IMPACT OF SUDDEN CARDIAC DEATH IN HEART FAILURE

Cardiac death soon after symptom onset - termed sudden cardiac death - is a major health problem. It is the commonest mode of death in the developed world and causes approximately 100,000 adult deaths per year in the United Kingdom and four times that in the United States [2-4]. In patients who die within an hour of the onset of symptoms or during sleep, more than 90% will be due to cardiac arrhythmias [5], and most of these events are likely to be caused by potentially reversible ventricular tachyarrhythmias [6].

SCD is a major cause of mortality in heart failure irrespective of its aetiology. Early data concerning the importance of SCD in heart failure came from epidemiological studies. Among 652 members of the Framingham Heart Study who developed congestive heart failure, 5-year survival rates after disease onset were 25% in men and 38% in women, and up to half of these deaths were sudden [7,8]. These findings still hold despite contemporary management. Mozaffarian et al assessed the mode of death in 10,538 ambulatory patients with New York Heart Association class II-IV heart failure enrolled in 6 randomised trials or registries [9]. Ischaemic heart disease accounted for 62% of cases. During 16,735 person-years of follow-up, 2014 deaths occurred, including 1014 sudden deaths and 684 pump-failure deaths. Though overall sudden death was the commonest mode of death, pump-failure was more frequent in advanced heart failure. Solomon et al studied 14,609 patients with asymptomatic left ventricular dysfunction or heart failure after myocardial infarction [10]. Over a median follow-up of 180 days there were 1067 cardiac arrests, 903 leading to death, which accounted for approximately a third of all deaths.

THE PATHOPHYSIOLOGY OF SUDDEN CARDIAC DEATH IN HEART FAILURE

Most cases of SCD in heart failure result from a malignant ventricular arrhythmia, either ventricular fibrillation or ventricular tachycardia [11]. This is supported by data from patients dying suddenly while undergoing Holter recording. In 157 episodes of SCD in ambulatory patients undergoing monitoring, 84% were secondary to ventricular arrhythmias, most commonly ventricular fibrillation (62%), while bradycardias accounted for only 16%

[12]. Though these were not exclusively patients with heart failure, it is probable that the mechanisms in heart failure are similar.

The underlying electrophysiological and molecular processes that lead to these malignant arrhythmias are incompletely understood. However there is likely to be a complex interplay between acquired abnormalities of cardiac structure and function, and genetic predisposition. The acquired changes include alterations in myocardial repolarisation, calcium homeostasis and neurohormonal signalling [13-15]. Two of the more important processes are action potential prolongation, due to changes in ion channel expression, and alterations in neurohormonal signalling.

Action Potential Prolongation and Ion Channel Expression

Prolongation of the action potential (AP) is a consistent finding in the ventricular myocardium of failing hearts irrespective of the cause [16]. The underlying physiological basis of the changes in AP duration is alteration in the functional expression of ion channel proteins, including potassium and sodium channels. The ventricular myocardium has a number of distinct classes of voltage-gated potassium ion channels. The most consistent finding in human and animal heart failure models is the downregulation of the I_{to} protein, but changes in the potassium channels I_{Kr} and I_{Ks} have also been noted [17-19]. Furthermore the importance of different potassium channels may vary depending on the aetiology of the heart failure [20]. Changes in sodium channels, which are important in the maintenance of the plateau phase of the action potential, have also been implicated [21].

The AP prolongation that occurs as a result of these changes in ion channel expression is inhomogeneous, leading to spatial and temporal heterogeneity in ventricular repolarisation [22]. It is this dispersion of repolarisation that may provide the substrate for the occurrence of malignant ventricular arrhythmias that lead to SCD [23]. These changes in repolarisation can be detected on the surface electrocardiogram (ECG), and form the basis of the risk stratification test Microvolt T-wave Alternans described below [24].

Altered Neurohormonal Signalling

Abnormal neurohormonal activation plays an integral role in the genesis of ventricular arrhythmias. Although the exact details of altered neurohormonal signalling are debated there is widespread acceptance of the importance of the autonomic nervous system and the renin-angiotensin-aldosterone (RAAS) system. Modulation of these neurohormonal systems have been shown to improve prognosis in patients with heart failure, including sudden death, and therapies that target them are now the mainstay of treatment for heart failure [25]. Further evidence of the importance of the sympathetic nervous system comes from the observation that there is a circadian variation in the frequency of SCD [26].

Myocardial infarction leads to sympathetic dennervation in the infarct zone [27]. This may be followed by neurilemma cell proliferation and axonal regeneration (nerve sprouting) leading to increased sympathetic nerve density or hyperinnervation in some areas of the myocardium [28]. In the normal human ventricle sympathetic activation causes a reduction in the action potential duration and a decrease in the dispersion of repolarisation [29]. In the failing heart the juxtaposition of dennervated and hyperinnervated myocardium may lead to spatial heterogeneity in ventricular repolarisation during sympathetic activation, predisposing to ventricular arrhythmogenesis [28]. Measuring these alterations in autonomic function has been demonstrated to be predictive of SCD, though such tests are not currently in widespread clinical use.

The RAAS system, through its two main effectors angiotensin II and aldosterone, has a range of effects on the myocardium that may predispose to malignant arrhythmias. These include induction of myocardial hypertrophy, increased collagen synthesis, promotion of inflammation and thrombosis, and modulation of active membrane properties [13].

Genetic Predisposition

Evidence for genetic predisposition to SCD comes from epidemiological data. Jouven et al assessed the occurrence of SCD in 7746 middle-aged men in the Paris Prospective Study. The risk of sudden death was increased by 80% in men who had a parental history of SCD, and nearly 9 times with a history in both parents [30].

It is well established that mutations in genes coding for cardiac ion channels underlie a range of heritable conditions that predispose to ventricular arrhythmias and SCD, including Long QT and Brugada syndrome [31]. It is also becoming clear that some gene polymorphisms, while not causing monogenic inherited arrhythmogenic syndromes, can increase susceptibility to proarrhythmic drugs by reducing "repolarisation reserve" [32]. It may be that specific polymorphisms in cardiac ion channel genes similarly predispose patients with heart failure to arrhythmias.

IMPLANTABLE CARDIOVERTER DEFIBRILLATORS

Since their introduction in the 1980s ICDs have revolutionised the management of patients at high risk of SCD. Multiple large randomised controlled trials have demonstrated that ICDs reduce mortality from SCD in high risk patients [33]. They are currently given to two groups of patients: survivors of life-threatening arrhythmias (secondary prevention) and patients at high risk for developing a life-threatening arrhythmia (primary prevention). In both of these settings they are both highly efficacious and cost effective [11,34].

Despite considerable effort to improve the results of out-of-hospital cardiac arrest, survival remains relatively low. Annual survival rates to hospital discharge of out-of-hospital cardiac arrest secondary to ventricular fibrillation are between 24% and 33% [35]. The use of ICDs for primary prevention of SCD is therefore of paramount importance in reducing overall SCD rates. In this respect the key issue is risk stratifying patients for SCD to identify which groups are at highest risk. While selecting patients for a secondary prevention ICD is relatively straightforward, identifying patients for primary prevention device therapy is more difficult.

TRADITIONAL RISK STRATIFICATION TOOLS TO GUIDE PRIMARY PREVENTION ICD USE

Risk stratification has been studied primarily in patients with congestive heart failure (CHF) or asymptomatic left ventricular dysfunction, as these groups are well known to be at increased risk of SCD. A large number of tests have been evaluated. These include tests of left ventricular function, autonomic function, ventricular repolarisation, and the presence or absence of spontaneous or inducible ventricular arrhythmias. The diverse nature of these tests reflects the complex underlying pathophysiology of ventricular arrhythmogenesis. The clinically relevant risk stratification tests are:

Left Ventricular Ejection Fraction (LVEF)

Depressed LVEF, as measured by echocardiography, contrast and radionuclide ventriculography, or magnetic resonance imaging, has long been recognised to be the most important determinant of all-cause mortality in patients with IHD [36,37]. More recently, a reduced LVEF has been demonstrated to be consistently the strongest predictor of SCD in both ischaemic and non-ischaemic cardiomyopathy.

In 14,609 post-MI patients enrolled in the VALIANT trial, depressed LVEF was the most powerful predictor of SCD [10]. In the first 30 days following MI each decrease in 5 percentage points in LVEF was associated with a 21 percent increase in the risk of sudden death or cardiac arrest with resuscitation. In a prospective study of 343 patients with idiopathic dilated cardiomyopathy, LVEF was the only significant predictor of arrhythmic events in multivariate analysis, with a relative risk of 2.3 per 10% decrease in ejection fraction [38].

As a result of this robust data a depressed LVEF has been the main entry criterion used in the randomised controlled clinical trials of primary prevention ICD therapy in heart failure [39,40].

Ambulatory Monitoring

A number of studies have suggested an association between the presence of non-sustained ventricular tachycardia (NSVT) on ambulatory monitoring and SCD in both ischaemic and non-ischaemic cardiomyopathy [41-43] However, although it is used as an important determinant in the latest UK NICE guidance on ICD use, more recent evidence has cast doubt on its predictive accuracy in the modern era [34,44].

Electrophysiological Studies (EPS)

Following the finding that post-MI patients with inducible ventricular arrhythmias had a significantly increased risk of SCD, EPS was for a long time considered the "gold standard" SCD risk stratification test in IHD patients [45-47]. However more recent studies have suggested that non-inducible patients are still at high risk of SCD, casting doubt on the prognostic value of EPS in IHD [48,49]. EPS has no significant prognostic role in non-ischaemic cardiomyopathy [50,51].

Microvolt T-wave Alternans (MTWA)

The electrocardiogram, or ECG, is a surface recording of the electrical activity of the heart. It records both ventricular depolarisation (the QRS complex) and repolarisation (the T-wave). Abnormalities in ventricular repolarisation, which are integral to arrhythmogenesis, are reflected in changes in the shape and size of the T-wave.

MTWA, which is a change in the size or shape of the T-wave on alternate beats, can be detected by complex computerised techniques. Multiple trials have demonstrated that MTWA testing is predictive of malignant arrhythmias. A meta-analysis of 19 studies, evaluating MTWA in 2608 patients over an average of 21 months follow-up, found a positive predictive value of 19.3% and negative predictive value of 97.2% [52]. There was no difference in predictive value between ischaemic and nonischaemic heart failure subgroups. However, patients with an indeterminate result were excluded from the analysis, and the high proportion of such patients (20-40%) is a significant limitation of MTWA. In addition there are currently a lack of prospective trials in which MTWA has been used to guide ICD use, and both of these issues will need addressing before MTWA is in routine clinical use [53].

Other Tests

In addition a number of other risk stratification tests have some predictive ability though they are not in widespread clinical use. These include tests of autonomic function, the signal-averaged ECG, and changes in the ECG QT segment [6].

Overall LVEF is consistently the strongest and most widely used predictor of SCD and the role of additional tests is currently unclear. Most contemporary guidelines suggest that heart failure patients with severely depressed LVEF (<30-35%) should be considered for an ICD without the need for additional testing, while patients with higher ejection fractions may benefit from further evaluation with additional risk stratification tests prior to ICD implantation [11,34].

THE LIMITATIONS OF CURRENT RISK STRATIFICATION SYSTEMS

Despite their proven benefits and universal recommendation in national and international guidelines [11,34 ,54], uptake of ICDs has been variable, and the majority of patients who might benefit from a device for 'primary prevention' of SCD do not receive one [55-58]. The reasons for this under-use are likely multifactorial. Firstly, implanted ICDs are often unused. Four year follow-up in two large trials, MADIT-II and SCD-HeFT, which used contemporary risk stratification tools to direct device use, showed under 40% of patients with ICDs received appropriate anti-tachycardic therapy [39,40]. Secondly, serious device-associated complications such as inappropriate device therapy and infection, though uncommon in trials, are increasingly recognised in routine practice [55,59 ,60]. Thirdly, at an estimated cost of £20102 per device, ICDs are an expensive technology [61,62].

The development of more accurate risk stratification systems would enable better targeting of ICD use. This would ensure devices are used in patients most likely to benefit and avoided in those who are unlikely to benefit but may still have complications. There is therefore significant value in developing improved risk stratification systems using existing and/or novel markers of SCD.

SERUM BIOMARKERS IN CARDIAC DISEASE

There has been a wealth of interest over the last decade in the use of biomarkers in cardiac disease. Many individual biomarkers have demonstrated associations with adverse cardiovascular outcomes, including C-reactive protein (CRP), interleukin-6, fibrinogen, d-dimer, albuminuruia, and plasminogen activator inhibitor type 1 [63-66]. Supported by systematic reviews confirming their value and consensus recommendations supporting their use, two specific serum markers, cardiac troponin (cTn) and brain natriuretic peptide (BNP), are now in widespread clinic use [68-71].

There is some evidence combining multiple cardiac biomarkers improves outcome prediction [72-74], though the magnitude of benefit is uncertain. For example, Wang et al studied 10 biomarkers, including CRP and BNP, in 3209 people in the Framingham Heart Study over 7 years and reported high "multimarker" scores increased the risks of death (hazard ratio 4.08) and major cardiovascular events (hazard ratio 1.84) [72]. However, they also noted that adding multimarker scores to conventional risk factors delivered only small increases in risk classification.

SERUM BIOMARKERS IN HEART FAILURE

Evidence of the value of serum biomarkers to predict SCD in heart failure comes from two types of study. Firstly, studies that have evaluated the relationship of biomarker levels to overall mortality or sudden cardiac death in heart failure. Secondly, studies that have evaluated biomarkers in patients with ICDs, using malignant ventricular arrhythmias as surrogate markers of SCD.

Serum Biomarkers to Predict Overall Mortality in Heart Failure

Heart failure is a clinical syndrome associated with complex molecular, endocrine and inflammatory changes [75]. The prognostic value of numerous serum biomarkers that reflect these underlying pathophysiological processes have been evaluated. Markers of neurohormonal activation, myocyte injury, myocardial stretch, and inflammation have all shown to be predictive of adverse outcomes [76].

Multiple studies have demonstrated that levels of serum inflammatory cytokines predict long-term heart failure mortality [77-79]. Rauchaus et al prospectively evaluated the predictive value of inflammatory cytokine levels in 152 patients with heart failure (121 patients in NYHA class II-III) [78]. During a mean 34 months follow-up there were 62 deaths. In univariate analyses tumour necrosis factor-alpha (TNF-α) and soluble TNF-receptors 1 and 2 (sTNF-R1/sTNFR2) (p<0.0001), interleukin-6 (p=0.005), and soluble

CD14 receptors (p=0.0007) were all predictive of death. In multivariate analysis the strongest predictor was sTNF-R2 (p<0.001), which proved better than depressed LVEF. Serum cardiac troponin (cTn) is also an independent predictor of adverse outcomes, including mortality, in both stable and decompensated heart failure [80-81].

The majority of these studies were small and evaluated the relationship of biomarkers to overall mortality rather than SCD. However the commonest mode of death in all but the most advanced heart failure is sudden death [9]. Therefore it is probable that these biomarkers predict SCD as well as overall mortality. This is supported by data from the VEST trial [79].

Deswal et al analysed circulating levels of two inflammatory cytokines (TNF and IL-6) and their cognate receptors in 1200 patients enrolled in a multicentre placebo-controlled trial of Vesnarinone, an inotropic drug, in advanced heart failure [79]. All patients were NYHA class III-IV and the aetiology of heart failure in the majority was IHD (58%). In the placebo group (384 patients) there were 65 deaths, 31 each due to SCD and pump failure. Data from these 384 patients demonstrated serum levels of tumor necrosis factor (p=0.02), IL-6 (p=0.002), sTNF-R1 (p=0.0001), and sTNF-R2 (p=0.0001) were all independent predictors of overall mortality in multivariate analysis. Although the predictive relationship of biomarkers to SCD was not specifically evaluated, levels of TNF and IL-6 were not significantly different between the SCD and pump failure groups.

Serum Biomarkers to Predict Sudden Cardiac Death in Heart Failure

The value of serum biomarkers to predict SCD in heart failure has been specifically evaluated in two prospective studies (Table 1) [83,84]. One enrolled patients with chronic heart failure of ischaemic and non-ischaemic aetiology [83], and the other post-MI patients [84]. Both demonstrated a significant association between a single serum biomarker measurement and subsequent SCD risk.

Berger et al examined the association of 4 serum biomarkers - BNP, N-terminal BNP (NT-BNP), N-terminal atrial natriuretic peptide (NT-ANP), and big endothelin - with SCD in 452 ambulatory patients with heart failure and LVEF <35% [83]. The aetiology of heart failure in the majority of these patients (65%) was non-ischaemic. During follow-up (592+/-387 days) there were 89 deaths of which 44 were sudden. Using univariate analyses the only significant predictors of sudden death were log BNP (p=0.0006), log N-ANP (p=0.0028), LVEF (p=0.0054), log N-BNP (p=0.0057), systolic blood pressure (p=0.0138), big endothelin (p=0.0326), and NYHA class (p=0.0375). However in multivariate analysis only log BNP (p=0.0006) was still significantly associated with SCD. The use of specific cardiac medication including beta-blockers, ACE-I and amiodarone, as well as the presence of IHD and diabetes, were not predictive of SCD.

Tapanainen et al prospectively evaluated the accuracy of plasma ANP, N-ANP, BNP and depressed LVEF in predicting SCD in 521 survivors of acute MI [84]. During a mean follow-up of 43 +/-13 months there were 33 deaths of which 16 were due to SCD. In univariate analysis, BNP (relative risk 4.4, p=0.011), ANP (RR 4.1, p=0.014) and N-ANP (RR 3.4, p=0.018) had similar accuracy as LVEF (RR 4.9, p=0.013) in predicting SCD. In multivariate analysis, after adjusting for clinical variables, only elevated BNP (p = 0.02) and low LVEF (<40%) (p = 0.03) remained as significant predictors of SCD. It should be noted that there was a high use of contemporary post-MI medical therapy in the cohort, including 97% beta-blockade.

Serum Biomarkers to Predict ICD Discharges

Implantable cardioverter defibrillators are extremely effective in terminating episodes of ventricular fibrillation (VF) and ventricular tachycardia (VT) that may otherwise have led to SCD. Therefore evaluating the relationship of biomarkers to SCD in patients with ICDs is potentially difficult. In addition to this therapeutic role however, ICDs also accurately record the occurrence of these malignant arrhythmias and the treatment given by the device, termed anti-tachycardic therapy. Thus the incidence of potentially life-threatening arrhythmias, as determined by device interrogation, may be used as a surrogate marker of SCD in these patients.

The ability of a range of serum biomarkers to predict malignant arrhythmias in ICD recipients has been assessed in 8 studies, enrolled 890 patients (Table 2) [85-91]. These studies, 6 of which were prospective, enrolled patients with both ischaemic and non-ischaemic heart failure. All but one study found biomarkers were able to predict the occurrence of malignant ventricular arrhythmias. The only study with negative findings was small and examined only 50 patients over 6 months [92].

Table 1. Studies evaluating the association of serum biomarkers with sudden cardiac death in patients with heart failure or left ventricular dysfunction

Study	Year	No. of patients	Aetiology of heart disease	Biomarkers	Results
Berger et al.	2002	452	IHD, NICM	BNP, NT-BNP, NT-ANP, big endothelin	All 4 biomarkers predictive of SCD in univariate analysis On multivariate analysis only BNP predictive
Tapanainen et al.	2004	521	IHD	BNP, ANP, NT-ANP	All 3 biomarkers predictive of SCD in univariate analysis On multivariate analysis only ANP and BNP predictive

IHD, ischaemic heart disease; NICM, non-ischaemic cardiomyopathy; BNP, brain natriuretic peptide; NT-BNP, N-terminal brain natriuretic peptide; NT-ANP, N-terminal atrial natriuretic peptide; ANP, atrial natriuretic peptide.

Table 2. Studies evaluating the association of serum biomarkers with malignant ventricular arrhythmias in ICD recipients.

Study	Year	No. of patients	Aetiology of heart disease	Biomarkers	End-point	Results
Manios et al [17]	2005	35	IHD	NT-proBNP	Appropriate device therapy for VT/VF	NT-proBNP predictive
Verma et al. [16]	2006	345	IHD, NICM	BNP, CRP	Appropriate device therapy for VT/VF	BNP predictive CRP not predictive
Biasucci et al [21]	2006	65	IHD	CRP	Appropriate device therapy for VT/VF	CRP predictive
Klingenberg et al [20]	2006	50	IHD	NT-proBNP	Appropriate device therapy for VT/VF	NT-proBNP predictive
Christ et al	2007	123	IHD, NICM	BNP	Appropriate device therapy for VT/VF, death or heart transplantation	BNP predictive
Yu et al [19]	2007	99	IHD	NT-proBNP	Appropriate device therapy for VT/VF	NT-proBNP predictive EPS not predictive
Blaney et al [18]	2007	121	IHD	PINP, PIIINP, TIMP1, BNP, CRP	Appropriate device therapy for VT/VF	All markers predictive
Konstantino et al	2007	50	IHD, NICM	BNP, CRP, IL-6, TNF-α	Appropriate device therapy for VT/VF	No markers predictive

IHD, ischaemic heart disease; NICM, non-ischaemic cardiomyopathy; BNP, brain natriuretic peptide; CRP, C-reactive protein; NT-proBNP, N-terminal pro-brain natriuretic peptide; PINP procollagen type I aminoterminal peptide; PIIINP, procollagen type III aminoterminal peptide, TIMP1, membrane metalloproteinase I; IL-6, interleukin 6; TNF-α, tumour necrosis factor alpha; VT, ventricular tachycardia; VF, ventricular fibrillation.

Six studies have investigated BNP (or N-terminal pro-BNP) and demonstrated it independently predicts malignant arrhythmias in patients with ICDs [85-90]. Three of the larger studies reported patients with BNP levels over the 50th centile had significantly more malignant arrhythmias (risk ratios between 2.2 and 3.8) [86,88 ,89]. Multivariate regression analyses in these studies examining traditional clinical and echocardiographic risk factors for SCD, found BNP most strongly predicted malignant arrhythmias and performed better than reduced LVEF.

Two studies investigated a broader range of serum biomarkers. Blangy et al prospectively evaluated markers of cardiac fibrosis [procollagen type I aminoterminal peptide (PINP), procollagen type III aminoterminal peptide (PIIINP), membrane metalloproteinase I (TIMP1)], myocardial pressure overload [brain natriuretic peptide (BNP)] and inflammation [high sensitivity (hs)-C-reactive protein] [88]. They observed 121 patients with IHD over 12 months. During this time 38 patients had appropriate device therapy for VT. In a multivariate analysis, LVEF <0.35 (OR = 2.19, P = 0.049), an increased serum BNP (OR = 3.75, P = 0.014), an increased hs-C-reactive protein (OR = 3.2, P = 0.006), an increased PINP (OR = 3.71, P = 0.009), and a decreased PIIINP (OR = 0.21, P = 0.003) were associated with a higher VT incidence. Biasucci et al studied 65 patients and confirmed the association with hsCRP [91].

One study has compared the predictive value of N-terminal pro-BNP (NT-pro-BNP) to the gold-standard of EPS [89]. Yu et al prospectively studied 99 patients with ICDs for prevention of SCD following MI. EPS and measurement of NT-pro-BNP were performed at study entry. During a mean follow-up of 556 (+/-122) days 23 patients received appropriate device therapy for VF/VT. On multivariate Cox regression analysis, only NT–pro-BNP level at or greater than median (497 ng/L) was a significant predictor for VT/VF occurrence (p=0.047). Neither univariate or multivariate analysis demonstrated any relationship between inducibility at EPS and the study end-points.

Table 3. Biomarkers demonstrated to predict the occurrence of sudden cardiac death or ventricular arrhythmias in patients with heart failure

Biomarker	Role of biomarker	No. of studies	Aetiology of heart failure in studies
Brain Natriuretic Peptide (BNP)	A natriuretic peptide largely released from the ventricles, in response to increases in intraventricular pressure and myocardial stretch	6	IHD, NICM
N-terminal pro Brain Natriuretic Peptide (NT-proBNP)	An N-terminal fragment that is co-secreted with BNP	3	IHD, NICM
Atrial Natriuretic Peptide (ANP)	A natriuretic peptide largely released from the atria in response to increases in intraatrial pressure and stretch	1	IHD
N-terminal Atrial Natriuretic Peptide (NT-ANP)	An N-terminal fragment that is co-secreted with ANP	2	IHD, NICM
C-reactive protein (CRP)	An acute phase reactant marker of systemic inflammation	3	IHD, NICM
Big endothelin	A precursor to endothelin, a vasoactive peptide involved in vascular homeostasis	1	IHD, NICM
Procollagen type I aminoterminal peptide	A marker of collagen turnover and myocardial fibrosis	1	IHD
Procollagen type III aminoterminal peptide	A marker of collagen turnover and myocardial fibrosis	1	IHD
Membrane metalloproteinase I	A marker of extracellular matrix remodelling	1	IHD

IHD, ischaemic heart disease; NICM, non-ischaemic cardiomyopathy.

SERUM BIOMARKERS TO GUIDE ICD USE?

Multiple studies have demonstrated that serum biomarkers can accurately predict adverse outcomes in patients with heart failure and asymptomatic left ventricular dysfunction of both ischaemic and non-ischaemic aetiology. A range of biomarkers predict both the occurrence of SCD in patients without ICDs and the occurrence of malignant arrhythmias in patients with devices (Table 3). In these studies individual biomarkers are at least as good as the current best marker of SCD risk, depressed LVEF. In the only trial to compare biomarkers to electrophysiological testing, serum NT-BNP was considerably more accurate than EPS in predicting malignant arrhythmias [89].

As predictive tests, biomarkers have significant advantages over current tools. Assessment of LVEF can be expensive, if performed by the gold-standard magnetic resonance imaging, and inaccurate, if performed using two-dimensional transthoracic echocardiography. EPS is expensive, invasive, associated with small but important risks to the patient, and often only available in larger cardiac centres. Ambulatory monitoring, to look for spontaneous ventricular arrhythmias, is not particularly reproducible [93]. In contrast, biomarker measurement is simple, relatively inexpensive, reproducible, and without direct patient risk.

The genesis of ventricular arrhythmias that lead to SCD is a complex process requiring the presence of both an abnormal myocardial substrate, needed to initiate and sustain an arrhythmia, and pro-arrhythmic triggers [11]. A range of electrophysiological and molecular alterations contribute to arrhythmogenesis in the failing heart, including changes in ion channel expression and neurohormonal modulation, and serum biomarkers may provide an assessment of these various processes. It is likely that optimal SCD risk stratification will require the combination of multiple tests that reflect these diverse upstream processes. As such the greatest potential benefit of biomarkers may be in measuring multiple complementary markers that assess distinct aspects of arrhythmic risk, or in combining biomarkers with traditional risk stratification tools. Currently there have been no studies evaluating this.

CONCLUSION

Despite the availability of a number of well characterised tests, risk stratification of SCD in patients with heart failure is currently sub-optimal.

The value of serum biomarkers in cardiovascular disease is well established. There is increasing data to suggest that individual serum biomarkers predict SCD at least as well as established risk stratification tools in heart failure patients. Biomarkers are available that provide an assessment of the diverse pathophysiological processes that are central to ventricular arrhythmogenesis, including myocardial stretch, inflammation, and neurohormonal activation. There is therefore significant need for further studies to evaluate the potential role of biomarkers, individually or in combination, in patient selection for ICDs.

References

[1]   Rosamond, W; Flegal, K; Friday, G; et al; American Heart Association Statistics Committee and Stroke Statistics Subcommittee. Heart disease and stroke statistics--2007 update: a report from the American Heart Association Statistics Committee and Stroke Statistics Subcommittee. *Circulation,* 2007, 115, e69-171.

[2]   Morgan Sudden cardiac death: opportunities for prevention. *Heart,* 2006, 92, 721-3.

[3]   Zipes, DP; Wellens, HJJ. Sudden cardiac death. *Circulation,* 1998, 98, 2334-51.

[4]   Zheng, ZJ; Croft, JB; Giles, EH; et al. Sudden cardiac death in the United States, 1989-1998. *Circulation,* 2001, 104, 2158-63.

[5]   Hinkle, LE; Jr, Thaler, HT. Clinical classification of cardiac deaths. *Circulation,* 1982, 65, 456-64.

[6]   Kusmirek, SL; Gold, MR. Sudden cardiac death: the role of risk stratification. *Am Heart J,* 2007, 153, (4 Suppl), 25-33.

[7]   Ho, KKL; Anderson, KM; Kannel, WB; et al. Survival after the onset of congestive heart failure in Framingham Heart Study subjects. *Circulation,* 1993, 88, 107-115.

[8]   Kannel, WB; Plehn, JF; Cupples, LA. Cardiac failure and sudden death in the Framingham Study. *Am Heart J,* 1988, 115, 869-75.

[9]   Mozaffarian, D; Anker, SD; Anand, I; et al. Prediction of mode of death in heart failure: the Seattle Heart Failure Model. *Circulation,* 2007, 116, 392-8.

[10] Solomon, S; Zelenkofske, S; McMurray, JJV; et al. Sudden death inpatients with myocardial infarction and left ventricular dysfunction, heart failure, or both. *N Engl J Med.*, 2005, 352, 2581 - 8.

[11] ACC/AHA/ESC 2006 Guidelines for Management of Patients With Ventricular Arrhythmias and the Prevention of Sudden Cardiac Death: a report of the American College of Cardiology/American Heart Association Task Force and the European Society of Cardiology Committee for Practice Guidelines (writing committee to develop Guidelines for Management of Patients With Ventricular Arrhythmias and the Prevention of Sudden Cardiac Death): developed in collaboration with the European Heart Rhythm Association and the Heart Rhythm Society. *Circulation,* 2006, 114,385-484.

[12] Bayes De Luna, A; Coumel, P; Leclercq, JF. Ambulatory sudden cardiac death: mechanisms of production of fatal arrhythmia on the basis of data from 157 cases. *Am Heart J,* 1989, 117, 151-9.

[13] Tomaselli, GF; Zipes, DP. What causes sudden death in heart failure? *Circ Res.,* 2004, 95, 754-63.

[14] Zipes, DP; Rubart, M. Neural modulation of cardiac arrhythmias and sudden cardiac death. *Heart Rhythm.* 2006, 3, 108-13.

[15] Rubart, M; Zipes, DP. Genes and cardiac repolarization: the challenge ahead. *Circulation,* 2005, 112, 1242-4.

[16] Tomaselli, GF; Marban, E. Electrophysiological remodeling in hypertrophy and heart failure. *Cardiovasc Res.,* 1999, 42, 270-283.

[17] Beuckelmann, DJ; Nabauer, M; Erdmann, E. Alterations of K currents in isolated human ventricular myocytes from patients with terminal heart failure. *Circ Res.,* 1993, 73, 379-385.

[18] Kaab, S; Nuss, HB; Chiamvimonvat, N; et al. Ionic mechanism of action potential prolongation in ventricular myocytes from dogs with pacing-induced heart failure. *Circ Res.,* 1996, 78, 262-273.

[19] Tsuji, Y; Opthof, T; Kamiya, K; et al. Pacing-induced heart failure causes a reduction of delayed rectifier potassium currents along with decreases in calcium and transient outward currents in rabbit ventricle. *Cardiovasc Res.,* 2000, 48, 300-309.

[20] Koumi, S; Backer, CL; Arentzen, CE. Characterization of inwardly rectifying K_ channel in human cardiac myocytes. Alterations in channel behavior in myocytes isolated from patients with idiopathic dilated cardiomyopathy. *Circulation,* 1995,92, 164-174.

[21] Undrovinas, AI; Maltsev, VA; Kyle, JW; et al. Gating of the late Na channel in normal and failing human myocardium. *J Mol Cell Cardiol,* 2002, 34, 1477-1489.

[22] Akar, FG; Rosenbaum, DS. Transmural electrophysiological heterogeneities underlying arrhythmogenesis in heart failure. *Circ Res.,* 2003, 93, 638-645.

[23] Weiss, J; Garfinkel, A; Karagueuzian, HS; et al. Chaos and the transition to ventricular fibrillation: a new approach to antiarrhythmic drug evaluation. *Circulation,* 1999, 99, 2819 -26.

[24] Narayan, SM. T-wave alternans and the susceptibility to ventricular arrhythmias. *J Am Coll Cardiol.,* 2006, 47, 269-81.

[25] ACC/AHA 2005 Guideline Update for the Diagnosis and Management of Chronic Heart Failure in the Adult: a report of the American College of Cardiology/American Heart Association Task Force on Practice Guidelines (Writing Committee to Update the 2001 Guidelines for the Evaluation and Management of Heart Failure): developed in collaboration with the American College of Chest Physicians and the International Society for Heart and Lung Transplantation: endorsed by the Heart Rhythm Society. *Circulation,* 2005, 112, e154-235.

[26] Muller, JE; Ludmer, PL; Willich, SN; et al. Circadian variation in the frequency of sudden cardiac death. *Circulation,* 1987, **75,** 131-138.

[27] Barber, MJ; Mueller, TM; Davies, BG; et al. Interruption of sympathetic and vagal-mediated afferent responses by transmural myocardial infarction. *Circulation,* 1985, 72, 623-631.

[28] Chen, LS; Zhou, S; Fishbein, MC; Chen, PS. New perspectives on the role of autonomic nervous system in the genesis of arrhythmias. *J Cardiovasc Electrophysiol,* 2007, 18, 123-7.

[29] Takei, M; Sasaki, Y; Yonezawa, T; et al. The autonomic control of the transmural dispersion of ventricular repolarization in anesthetized dogs. *J Cardiovasc Electrophysio,* 1999, 10, 981-989.

[30] Jouven, X; Desnos, M; Guerot, C; Ducimetière, P. Predicting sudden death in the population: the Paris Prospective Study I. *Circulation,* 1999, 99, 1978-83.

[31] Brugada, J; Brugada, R; Brugada, P. Channelopathies: a new category of diseases causing sudden death. *Herz,* 2007, 32, 185-91.

[32] Remme, CA; Bezzina, CR. Genetic modulation of cardiac repolarization reserve. *Heart Rhythm,* 2007, 4, 608-10.

[33] Ezekowitz, JA; Rowe, BH; Dryden, DM; et al. Systematic review: implantable cardioverter defibrillators for adults with left ventricular systolic dysfunction. *Ann Intern Med.*, 2007, 147, 251-62.

[34] TA95 Implantable cardioverter defibrillators for arrhythmias. http://guidance.nice.org.uk/TA95/guidance/pdf/English

[35] Cobb, LA; Weaver, WD; Fahrenbruch, CE; et al. Community-based interventions for sudden cardiac death. Impact, limitations, and changes. *Circulation,* 1992, 85, 98 -102.

[36] Multicenter Post Infarction Research Group. Risk Stratification and survival after myocardial infarction. *N Engl J Med.,* 1983, 309, 331-6.

[37] Nelson GR, Cohn PF, Gorlin R. Prognosis in medically-treated coronary artery disease: influence of ejection fraction compared to other parameters. *Circulation,* 1975, 52,408-12.

[38] Grimm, W; Christ, M; Bach, J; et al. Noninvasive arrhythmiarisk stratification in idiopathic dilated cardiomyopathy: results of the Marburg cardiomyopathy study. *Circulation,* 2003, 108, 2883-91.

[39] Bardy, GH; Lee, KL; Mark, DB; et al. Amiodarone or an implantable cardioverter-defibrillator for congestive heart failure. *N Engl J Med.,* 2005, 352, 225-37.

[40] Moss, AJ; Zareba, W; Hall, WJ; et al. Prophylactic implantation of a defibrillator in patients with myocardial infarction and reduced ejection fraction. *N Engl J Med.,* 2002, 346, 877 - 83.

[41] Anderson, KP; DeCamilla, J; Moss, AJ. Clinical significance of ventricular tachycardia (3 beats or longer) detected during ambulatory monitoring after myocardial infarction. *Circulation,* 1978, **57,** 890-7.

[42] Bigger, Jr JT; Fleiss, JL; Kleiger, R; et al. The relationships among ventricular arrhythmias, left ventricular dysfunction, and mortality in the 2 years after myocardial infarction. *Circulation,* 1984, 69, 250-8.

[43] Grimm, W; Christ, M; Maisch, B. Long runs of non-sustained ventricular tachycardia on 24-hour ambulatory electrocardiogram predict major arrhythmic events in patients with idiopathic dilated cardiomyopathy. *PACE,* 2005, 28, S207-10.

[44] Ma¨kikallio, TH; Barthel, P; Schneider, R; et al. Prediction of sudden cardiac death after acute myocardial infarction: role of Holter monitoring in the modern treatment era. *Eur Heart J,* 2005, 26, 762-9.

[45] Bourke, JP; Richards, DA; Ross, DL; et al. Routine programmed electrical stimulation in survivors of acute myocardial infarction for prediction of spontaneous ventricular tachyarrhythmias during follow-

up: results, optimal stimulation protocol and cost-effective screening. *J Am Coll Cardiol,* 1991, 18, 780-8.

[46] Iesaka, Y; Nogami, A; Aonuma, K; et al. Prognostic significance of sustained monomorphic ventricular tachycardia induced by programmed ventricular stimulation using up to triple extrastimuli in survivors of acute myocardial infarction. *Am J Cardiol,* 1990, 65, 1057- 63.

[47] Nogami, A; Aonuma, K; Takahashi, A; et al. Usefulness of early versus late programmed ventricular stimulation in acute myocardial infarction. *Am J Cardiol,* 1991, 68, 13-20.

[48] Daubert, JP; Zareba, W; Hall, WJ; et al. Predictive value of ventricular arrhythmia inducibility for subsequent ventricular tachycardia or ventricular fibrillation in Multicenter Automatic Defibrillator Implantation Trial (MADIT) II patients. *J Am Coll Cardiol,* 2006, 47, 98-107.

[49] Buxton, AE; Lee, KL; DiCarlo, L; et al. Electrophysiologic testing to identify patients with coronary artery disease who are at risk for sudden death. *N Engl J Med.,* 2000, 342, 1937-45.

[50] Poll, DS; Marchlinski, FE; Buxton, AE; et al. Usefulness of programmed stimulation in idiopathic dilated cardiomyopathy. *Am J Cardiol,* 1986, 58, 992-7.

[51] Meinertz, T; Treese, N; Kasper, W; et al. Determinants of prognosis in idiopathic dilated cardiomyopathy as determined by programmed electrical stimulation. *Am J Cardiol,* 1985, 56, 337-41.

[52] Gehi, AK; Stein, RH; Metz, LD; et al. Microvolt T-wave alternans for the risk stratification of ventricular tachyarrhythmic events a metaanalysis. *J Am Coll Cardiol,* 2005, 46, 75-82.

[53] Gold, MR; Spencer, W. T wave alternans for ventricular arrhythmia risk stratification. *Curr Opin Cardiol,* 2003, 18, 1-5.

[54] Al-Khatib, SM; Sanders, GD; Bigger, JT Preventing tomorrow's sudden cardiac death today: part I: Current data on risk stratification for sudden cardiac death. *Am Heart J,* 2007, 153, 941-50.

[55] Sanders, GD; Al-Khatib, SM; Berliner, E; et al; Expert panel participating in a Duke Center for the Prevention of Sudden Cardiac Death-sponsored conference Preventing tomorrow's sudden cardiac death today: part II: Translating sudden cardiac death risk assessment strategies into practice and policy. *Am Heart J,* 2007, 153, 951-9.

[56] Pacemakers and Implantable Defibrillators: A Two Year National Survey for 2003 and 2004. Network Devices Survey Group. http://www.devicesurvey.com/

[57] Scott, PA; Gorman, S; Andrews, NP, et al. Estimation of the requirement for implantable cardioverter defibrillators for the primary prevention of sudden cardiac death post-myocardial infarction based on UK national guidelines (2006) *Europace* 2008, 10, 453-7.

[58] Plummer, CJ; Irving, J; Mccomb, JM. The incidence of implantable cardioverter defibrillator indications in patients admitted to all coronary care units in a single district. *Europace,* 2005, **7,** 266-72.

[59] Reynolds, MR; Cohen, DJ; Kugelmass, AD; et al. The frequency and incremental cost of major complications among medicare beneficiaries receiving implantable cardioverter-defibrillators. *J Am Coll Cardiol,* 2006, 47, 2493-7.

[60] Gould, PA; Krahn, AD. Complications associated with implantable cardioverter-defibrillator replacement in response to device advisories. *JAMA,* 2006, 295, 1907-11.

[61] TA95 Arrhythmia - implantable cardioverter defibrillators (ICDs): *Analysis of cost impact.* http://guidance.nice.org.uk/TA95/costtemplate/xls/English

[62] Hlatky MA, Mark DB. The high cost of implantable defibrillators. *Eur Heart J,* 2007, 28, 388-91.

[63] Ridker, PM; Rifai, N; Stampfer, MJ; Hennekens, CH. Plasma concentration of interleukin-6 and the risk of future myocardial infarction among apparently healthy men. *Circulation,* 2000, 101, 1767-72.

[64] Danesh, J; Wheeler, JG; Hirschfield, GM; et al. C-reactive protein and other circulating markers of inf lammation in the prediction of coronary heart disease. *N Engl J Med.,* 2004, 350, 1387-97.

[65] Danesh, J; Lewington, S; Thompson, SG; et al. Plasma fibrinogen level and the risk of major cardiovascular diseases and nonvascular mortality: an individual participant meta-analysis. *JAMA,* 2005, 294, 1799-809.

[66] Cushman, M; Lemaitre, RN; Kuller, LH; et al. Fibrinolytic activation markers predict myocardial infarction in the elderly: the Cardiovascular Health Study. *Arterioscler Thromb Vasc Biol.,* 1999, 19, 493-8.

[67] Hoekstra, T; Geleijnse, JM; Schouten, EG; Kluft, C. Plasminogen activator inhibitor-type 1: its plasma determinants and relation with cardiovascular risk. *Thromb Haemost,* 2004, 91, 861-72.

[68] Doust, JA; Pietrzak, E; Dobson, A; Glasziou, P. How well does B-type natriuretic peptide predict death and cardiac events in patients with heart failure: systematic review. *BMJ,* 2005, 330, 625-8.

[69] Tang, WH; Francis, GS; Morrow, DA; et al; National Academy of Clinical Biochemistry Laboratory Medicine. National Academy of Clinical Biochemistry Laboratory Medicine practice guidelines: Clinical utilization of cardiac biomarker testing in heart failure. *Circulation,* 2007, 116, 99-109.

[70] The Joint ESC/ACC Committee. Myocardial infarction redefined-A consensus document of the Joint ESC/ACC Committee for the Redefinition of Myocardial Infarction. *Eur Heart J,* 2000, 21, 1502-1513.

[71] Wang, TJ; Larson, MG; Levy, D; et al. Plasma natriuretic peptide levels and the risk of cardiovascular events and death. *N Engl J Med.,* 2004, 350, 655-63.

[72] Wang, TJ; Gona, P; Larson, MG; et al. Multiple biomarkers for the prediction of first major cardiovascular events and death. *N Engl J Med.,* 2006, 355, 2631-9.

[73] Sabatine, MS; Morrow, DA; De Lemos, JA; et al. Multimarker approach to risk stratification in non-ST elevation acute coronary syndromes: simultaneous assessment of troponin I, C-reactive protein, and B-type natriuretic peptide. *Circulation,* 2002,105, 1760-3.

[74] Blankenberg, S; McQueen, MJ; Smieja, M; et al; HOPE Study Investigators. Comparative impact of multiple biomarkers and N-Terminal pro-brain natriuretic peptide in the context of conventional risk factors for the prediction of recurrent cardiovascular events in the Heart Outcomes Prevention Evaluation (HOPE) Study. *Circulation,* 2006 114, 201-8.

[75] Braunwald, E; Bristow, MR. Congestive heart failure: fifty years of progress. *Circulation,* 2000, 102, 14-23.

[76] De Virginy, DR. Novel and potential future biomarkers for assessment of the severity and prognosis of chronic heart failure : a clinical review. *Heart Fail Rev.,* 2006, 11, 333-4.

[77] Maeda, K; Tsutamoto, T; Wada, A; et al. High levels of plasma brain natriuretic peptide and interleukin-6 after optimized treatment for heart failure are independent risk factors for morbidity and mortality in patients with congestive heart failure. *J Am Coll Cardiol,* 2000, 36, 1587-93.

[78] Rauchhaus, M; Doehner, W; Francis, DP; et al. Plasma cytokine parameters and mortality in patients with chronic heart failure. *Circulation,* 2000, 102, 3060-7.

[79]   Deswal, A; Petersen, NJ; Feldman, AM; et al. Cytokines and cytokine receptors in advanced heart failure: an analysis of the cytokine database from the Vesnarinone trial (VEST). *Circulation,* 2001, 103, 2055-9

[80]   Sato, Y; Yamada, T; Taniguchi, R; et al. Persistently increased serum concentrations of cardiac troponin T in patients with idiopathic dilated cardiomyopathy are predictive of adverse outcomes. *Circulation,* 2001, 103, 369-374.

[81]   Horwich, TB; Patel, J; MacLellan, WR; Fonarow, GC. Cardiac troponin I is associated with impaired hemodynamics, progressive left ventricular dysfunction, and increased mortality rates in advanced heart failure. *Circulation,* 2003, 108, 833- 838.

[82]   Kuwabara, Y; Sato, Y; Miyamoto, T; et al. Persistently increased serum concentrations of cardiac troponin in patients with acutely decompensated heart failure are predictive of adverse outcomes. *Circ J.,* 2007, 71, 1047-51

[83]   Berger, R; Huelsman, M; Strecker, K; et al. B-type natriuretic peptide predicts sudden death in patients with chronic heart failure. *Circulation,* 2002, 105, 2392-7.

[84]   Tapanainen, JM; Lindgren, KS; Ma¨kikallio, TH; et al. Natriuretic peptides as predictors of non-sudden and sudden cardiac death after acute myocardial infarction in the beta-blocking era. *J Am Coll Cardiol,* 2004, 43, 757-63.

[85]   Christ, M; Sharkova, J; Bayrakcioglu, S; et al. B-type natriuretic peptide levels predict event-free survival in patients with implantable cardioverter defibrillators. *Eur J Heart Fail,* 2007, 9, 272-9.

[86]   Verma, A; Kilicaslan, F; Martin, DO; et al. Preimplantation B-type natriuretic peptide concentration is an independent predictor of future appropriate implantable defibrillator therapies. *Heart,* 2006, 92, 190-5.

[87]   Manios, EG; Kallergis, EM; Kanoupakis, EM; et al. Amino-terminal pro-brain natriuretic peptide predicts ventricular arrhythmogenesis in patients with ischemic cardiomyopathy and implantable cardioverter-defibrillators. *Chest.,* 2005, 128,2604-10.

[88]   Blangy, H; Sadoul, N; Dousset, B; et al. Serum BNP, hs-C-reactive protein, procollagen to assess the risk of ventricular tachycardia in ICD recipients after myocardial infarction. *Europace,* 2007, 9, 724-9.

[89]   Yu, H; Oswald, H; Gardiwal, A; et al. Comparison of N-terminal pro-brain natriuretic peptide versus electrophysiologic study for predicting future outcomes in patients with an implantable cardioverter defibrillator after myocardial infarction. *Am J Cardiol,* 2007, 100, 635-9.

[90] Klingenberg, R; Zugck, C; Becker, R; et al. Raised B-type natriuretic peptide predicts implantable cardioverter-defibrillator therapy in patients with ischaemic cardiomyopathy. *Heart,* 2006, 92, 1323-4.

[91] Biasucci, LM; Giubilato, G; Biondi-Zoccai, G; et al. C reactive protein is associated with malignant ventricular arrhythmias in patients with ischaemia with implantable cardioverter-defibrillator. *Heart,* 2006, 92, 1147-8.

[92] Konstantino, Y; Kusniec, J; Reshef, T; et al. Inflammatory biomarkers are not predictive of intermediate-term risk of ventricular tachyarrhythmias in stable CHF patients. *Clin Cardiol,* 2007, 30, 408-13.

[93] Senges, JC; Becker, R; Schreiner, KD; et al. Variability of Holter electrocardiographic findings in patients fulfilling the noninvasive MADIT criteria. Multicenter Automatic Defibrillator Implantation Trial. Pacing Clin Electrophysiol, 2002, 25, 183-90.

In: Heart Failure: Symptoms, Causes...   ISBN: 978-1-61668-959-9
Editor: Madison S. Wright, pp. 143-158 © 2010 Nova Science Publishers, Inc.

Chapter 9

CORONARY ARTERY BYPASS GRAFTING FOR CHRONIC AND ACUTE HEART FAILURE

Marco Pocar, Andrea Moneta, Davide Passolunghi,
Alessandra Di Mauro, Alda Bregasi, Roberto Mattioli
and Francesco Donatelli
Unit of Cardiac Surgery and Echo-Lab; Scientific Institute MultiMedica
Hospital; University of Milan; Milan, Italy

ABSTRACT

The techniques and reproducibility of surgical coronary revascularization rely on over forty-year experience. However, surgery for ischemic heart disease with associated left ventricular dysfunction carried high if not prohibitive operative risk during the pioneering and early era of coronary surgery. Although the benefits of revascularization in this context have been well documented, the propensity to operate on patients with heart failure still often relies on concurrent anginal symptoms. Similarly, many surgeons are reluctant to offer surgery aimed to reverse low cardiac output during acute or evolving myocardial infarction.

The purpose of this chapter is to depict up-to-date strategies and attitudes toward coronary operations in chronic or acute heart failure, focusing on personal experience with ischemic cardiomyopathy and acute coronary syndromes complicated by pump dysfunction or shock. Emphasis will be given to the selection of patients, evolving technology, technical strategies, and ultimately to the limitations of isolated coronary revascularization and the increasing role of associated surgical procedures in ischemic cardiomyopathy.

Coronary artery bypass grafting (CABG) relies on worldwide experience gained during over forty years since the first clinical successful series of patients [1]. In spite of technical reproducibility, low risks and predictable results, patients with associated left ventricular (LV) dysfunction carried a high if not prohibitive operative risk during the pioneering and early era of coronary surgery. Indications for CABG have broadened during the last two decades, but many institutions are still reluctant to offer surgery in higher-risk settings, namely, severely depressed systolic function, overt heart failure and acute coronary syndromes complicated by low cardiac output.

ISCHEMIC CARDIOMYOPATHY AND CHRONIC ISCHEMIC HEART FAILURE

The most common modality of cardiovascular death is refractory heart failure secondary to coronary artery disease. Although patients undergoing isolated CABG represent a lower-risk population among cardiac surgical candidates, LV dysfunction represents an independent risk factor for hospital and 30-day mortality. This is most often depicted by a poor LV ejection fraction (LVEF), particularly when lower than 30-35%, a higher New York Heart Association functional class or, even more dramatically, a low output state and the requirement for inotropic support, which all represent typical variables included in widely employed risk-scoring systems [2, 3]. Benefits of revascularization outweigh by far the risks of surgery in patients with LV dysfunction and concurrent angina pectoris, which traditionally underlies a potential for viability and thus for contractile recovery [4]. Conversely, indications for CABG in case of prevalent heart failure symptoms have been outlined more recently [5-7].

Indications for Revascularization

Selection of patients remains controversial, and is even more complex in the younger age group with advanced heart failure, which might be potentially considered for transplantation. However, good long-term survival, as late as 10-to-15 years after CABG, can be anticipated in selected subgroups of patients [7].

CORONARY TARGETS

The vast majority of patients with LV dysfunction considered for CABG have triple-vessel disease, whereas the severity and distribution of coronary atherosclerosis well correlates with LV dysfunction. The quality of distal coronary territories is an obvious issue and diffuse distal disease with poor peripheral run-off, which is worsened by higher intraventricular diastolic pressures, has been outlined as a strong pedictor of a poor outcome in these patients [6]. However, the definition of an unfavourable surgical anatomy cannot be standardized and must be judged on an individual basis. Furthermore, vascular wall remodeling has been outlined in experimental animals and may correlate with reduced perfusion after CABG [8]. As a general rule, more severe LV dysfunction implies more graftable targets, and more severe and proximal coronary stenoses as a pre-requisite to render CABG equally appealing. The best candidates are those presenting with left main or triple-vessel disease, severe and proximally-located stenoses, and undiseased distal branches.

MYOCARDIAL VIABILITY

Different imaging techniques may be employed for the detection and quantification of myocardial viability. These include single photon emission tomography, positron emission tomography, magnetic resonance imaging techniques, and echocardiography [9-13]. Stress-tests are often performed following inotrope infusion, typically dobutamine, or exercise. A detailed description of the single diagnostic tools is beyond the scope of this chapter, but the differentiation into viable and non-viable myocardium may not always be clear-cut. The degree of segmental viability is derived measuring respective uptake of specific tracers, which indicate a metabolic shift toward glucose consumption (positron emission tomography), the integrity of cellular and mitochondrial membranes (nuclear scintigraphy), or the amount of tissue fibrosis (magnetic resonance). Wall motion segmental assessment can also be performed with various techniques, but is more straighforward with echocardiography. The latter and magnetic resonance also allow the analysis of ventricular wall thickening during the cardiac cycle.

The detection of myocardial viability plays a substantial role not only in the stratification of operative risk, but also in the prediction of the probability of reverse LV remodeling, irrespective of associated angina [14]. Some institutions indicate CABG without preoperative viability testing [6], but the absence of akinetic and viable segments, commonly termed hibernating myocardium, correlates with a worse outcome. Particular efforts have been devoted to quantify the amount of hibernating myocardium to predict a successful operation and thus to serve as a reference for appropriate selection of patients. At the beginning of our experience in the late Eighties, screening for myocardial viability in angina-free patients was undertaken with positron emission tomography in case of LVEF < 40%, and CABG was planned on the basis of a minimum of 2 of 5 viable and akinetic segments (anterior, septal, apical, lateral, inferior) with critically stenotic coronary tributaries [7]. Nowadays, the LV is subdivided into the 16 segments which abitually serve for regional wall motion analysis at echocardiography, and the presence of a minimum of 4 akinetic and viable segments has been identified as a predictor of reverse LV remodeling after CABG. During decision making, however, the surgeon should keep in mind the limitations of isolated CABG in patients with more advanced cardiomyopathy. This point is discussed in a separate section.

Surgical Technique

Basic principles of CABG technique are well established, but specific aspects concerning myocardial protection, the choice of conduits and distal target vessels, and, ultimately, the decision whether to employ or not cardiopulmonary bypass are of utmost importance in case of LV dysfunction.

CARDIOPULMONARY BYPASS AND MYOCARDIAL PROTECTION

Although off-pump operations have been reported in patients with poor LVEF [15], displacement maneuvers or prolonged exposure of the lateral and posterior LV are undoubtedly less tolerated in case of dilated hearts. During off-pump operations patients are more prone to intraoperative hypotension or electrical instabilization, which may be as detrimental as ischemia-reperfusion injury due to conventional aortic cross-clamping and cardioplegia arrest. Furthermore, a lower patency rate of distal anastomoses and a reduced number of grafts-per-patient have been reported after off-pump operations when compared to conventional CABG [16], and this is likely to represent an even more critical issue in case of LV dysfunction. Thus, traditional CABG with extracorporeal circulation is the favored strategy at our institution. Operations are performed on moderately hypothermic (32-33 °C core temperature) cardiopulmonary bypass with blood antegrade and retrograde cardioplegia, normothermic induction, cold maintaining doses every 20 minutes, and substrate-enriched controlled reperfusion, following Buckberg's protocols for energy-depleted hearts [17]. The LV can be vented, typically through the right superior pulmonary vein, to prevent rewarming from extracoronary collateral blood flow during construction of the anastomoses or to avoid inadvertent LV distension, especially during the reperfusion phase, but this adjunct is generally unnecessary and is now seldom applied by our team. Unusual exceptions may include, for example, disturbing collateral flow obscuring the surgical field or mild aortic insufficiency. Finally, off-pump CABG is reserved to the rare occurrence of isolated revascularization in the left anterior descending (LAD) and proximal-to-mid right coronary territories, whereas beating-heart CABG with cardiopulmonary bypass support – i.e., conventional CABG without cardioplegia – can be an attractive alternative in the presence of a severely calcified ascending aorta. In the latter case, our preferred arterial cannulation site is the undersurface of the distal arch.

STRATEGY OF REVASCULARIZATION

The importance of complete revascularization cannot be overemphasized in patients with LV dysfunction. Our policy is to bypass all stenoses ≥50% on all technically graftable targets. In view of the high prevalence of triple-vessel disease in case of poor LV function, the majority of patients receive three or more distal bypass grafts. Bilateral internal thoracic artery (ITA) grafts are applied in as many as 50% of the patients and maintained pedicled whenever possible. Although this represents a debated issue, we believe this may be beneficial irrespectively of late outcome, when considering that distal run-off is often reduced in dilated hearts with higher filling pressures, particularly in the left coronary territories, and in branches supplying hibernating myocardium [18, 19]. Speculatively, this policy is likely to yield lower graft failure rates when compared to a traditional wider use of saphenous vein grafts. Consequently, we generally graft the left ITA to the LAD, avoiding sequential grafts on diagonal branches, and the right ITA to the circumflex territory with a course in the transverse sinus. ITAs (especially the right) are often harvested with a skeletonized technique. In case of inadequate right ITA length – a not infrequent occurrence when dealing with dilated hearts – conduits may be switched, i.e., grafting the right ITA to the LAD and the left ITA to the circumflex, thus avoiding free arterial grafts. In spite of a relatively low probability of reintervention in patients with poor LV function, this combination is generally avoided in patients younger than 65 years because of the obvious hazards of a right ITA-to-LAD graft crossing the midline between a dilated heart and the sternum. Alternatively, a dominant right coronary artery may be chosen as the target for the second ITA, even though grafts in this territory are most often constructed on the posterior descending branch. The remaining target vessels are bypassed with traditional saphenous vein grafts, which are usually constructed first. We often employ sequential venous grafts, provided that the caliber of the most distal target is not diminutive. Proximal anastomoses are completed during a single period of aortic cross-clamping, generally immediately after the corresponding distal anastomosis/-es, to ensure the widest possible delivery of cardioplegia during infusion of maintaining doses and, most importantly, during myocardial reperfusion and rewarming. In view of the potential hazards of spasm, which might be triggered by hypotension or, more in general, by perioperative instability, we do not favor alternative arterial grafts, such as the radial artery, in patients with LV dysfunction unless adequate veins are unavailable.

Intensive and Perioperative Care

Perioperative care, both before and after surgery, is of obvious importance in patients with LV dysfunction. When excluding acute coronary syndromes, intensive management is usually required only postoperatively in isolated CABG operations. Preoperative invasive hemodynamic monitoring with a Swan-Ganz catheter, inotropic pharmacologic support or aortic balloon counterpulsation may occasionally be indicated in decompensated patients. Nowadays, however, the latter are most often candidates for additional procedures, such as mitral or left ventricular restoration surgery.

Our policy is to employ inotropes and IABP preoperatively only in hemodynamically unstable patients. In rare instances, pre-treatment with intravenous levosimendan has been initiated 24 hours before surgery. With respect to the intraoperative and early postoperative course we usually employ low-dose dopamine ($\leq$ 6 mcg/Kg/min), epinephrine as a second-line inotropic agent, and phosphodiesterase inhibitors (milrinone) as additional resort. The theoretical advantage of milrinone is to improve contractility without a significant increase in myocardial oxygen consumption, whereas the combination of a different class of drugs allows a lower dose of catecholamines. Milrinone is generally associated when higher-dose epinephrine infusion rates ($\geq$ 0.08-0.1 mcg/Kg/min) are necessary. IABP is considered when low cardiac output ($< 2L/min/m^2$) persists in spite of multiple inotropes or, more rarely, in case of electrical instability. Most patients with severe LV dysfunction receive double arterial invasive monitoring – radial and femoral – before skin incision. This facilitates expeditious IABP insertion when needed. Finally, Swan-Ganz monitoring is seldom used in patients undergoing isolated CABG at our institution. Direct left atrial catheterization is sometimes used intraoperatively for temporary monitoring of left-sided filling pressures during weaning from cardiopulmonary bypass. All patients with ischemic LV dysfunction start medical heart failure therapy with ACE-inhibitors or anti-angiotensin receptor inhibitors, and beta-blockers as soon as possible, almost invariably before discharge from the intensive care unit.

Associated Procedures

Limitations of isolated CABG in patients with poor LV function are controversial and the attitude toward additional surgical procedures varies widely between institutions. It must be stressed that the vast majority of late deaths (> 80%) are cardiac-related, with progressive heart failure and sudden death as predominating causes, with a near-equal proportion [7]. In a minority of cases acute myocardial infarction is the modality of cardiac death during follow-up. In addition, other cardiovascular complications (neurologic, peripheral, renal) are the main cause of death in another subgroup of patients, most commonly in diabetics.

Our general policy has changed over time. Schematically, the essential points are addressed here:

1. Patients with a preoperative widened QRS complex are evaluated for LV dyssynchrony and functional mitral regurgitation at echocardiography, eventually with stress testing. In cases of widened QRS, an epicardial lead is implanted on the lateral LV wall and drawn subcutaneously to the left subclavicular region. This adds minimal surgical invasiveness to the operation and greatly facilitates subsequent resynchronization therapy. In addition, a temporary pacing wire may be connected to the permanent lead to allow perioperative atrio-biventricular pacing to improve cardiac output [20]. Similarly, indications for implantation of an automatic cardioverter defibrillator is evaluated in all patients with LV function.

2. The role of associated mitral valve surgery for functional insufficiency is a controversial issue, especially with respect to the potential for improved late survival [21-25]. However, the correlation between ischemic mitral regurgitation and reduced life expectancy in patients with coronary artery disease and prior myocardial infarction is well-established [26] and operative risk for associated undersized mitral annuloplasty appear to be low. As a consequence, we now tend to implant a prosthetic ring in the presence of moderate or severe mitral insufficiency.

3. An exaustive discussion regarding left ventricular reduction surgery is beyond the objectives of this chapter. However, a number of variables describing systolic or diastolic dysfunction, and correlated with the degree of LV remodeling have been recently outlined as independent predictors of late outcome in heart failure, including patients undergoing cardiac operations. The former include LV end-diastolic pressure, end-systolic volume index, atrial volume index and diastolic filling patterns [7, 27, 28]. In particular, LV end-systolic volume index is a resultant of cardiac dilatation and LVEF, and well depicts LV systolic dysfunction irrespective of the severity of associated mitral insufficiency. In this respect patients with an enlarged LV and previous are increasingly being scheduled for LV reconstruction, most often for the Dor procedure or LV restoration, in the presence of an LV end-systolic volume index > 45 or 50 mL/m^2. Ongoing trials will better define the respective benefits (and risks) of this approach.

HEART FAILURE AND CARDIOGENIC SHOCK IN ACUTE MYOCARDIAL INFARCTION

Since the early reports concerning CABG for acute coronary syndromes in the late Sixties [29], indications and results have been impressively influenced by the introduction of systemic thrombolysis, percutaneous coronary interventions (PCI) and coronary stenting in clinical practice. In parallel, revascularization performed within 4 to 6 hours from the onset of ischemia has been well correlated with a higher probability of survival and recovery of LV function [30]. Consequently, indications for CABG played a substantial part in the early era, but have been confined as a last-line resort with the progressive development of medical and interventional reperfusion strategies. However, mortality rates below 5% have been reported in randomized trials since the late Eighties when emergency CABG is indicated as first-choice option in non-selected patients [31].

Nowadays, indications for emergency CABG may vary considerably between institutions and are dictated not only by the general attitudes of a particular cardiovascular department and team but also by logistic problems, especially when transportation of an unstable patients is required. Surgery almost unvariably requires longer time intervals to achieve reperfusion and the availability of an invasive cardiology laboratory or cardiac surgical unit on site is a major determinant of clinical decision making in this setting. However, CABG offers the following advantages:

1. it allows complete revascularization in virtually all patients that could benefit from PCI or thrombolysis, and reduces 1-year mortality from 10% to 2-3% [32];
2. myocardial and end-organ protection and perfusion can be selectively applied with extracorporeal perfusion techniques;
3. in spite of suboptimal mortality rates, the two previous points renders surgsry as the preferred approach for patients with heart failure or in cardiogenic shock [33-34]. Importantly, pump failure is the most common modality of death in this population, whereas mortality approaches 100% in case of medical management of postinfarction cardiogenic shock.

Indications for Operation

Indications for CABG in acute myocardial infarction, other than failed PCI or postinfarction mechanical complications, are essentially dictated by the following variables:

1. Extent of myocardium at risk. It should be stressed that this issue pertains not only to the infarcted territory, but also to the remote myocardium. Longer intervals from onset of ischemia progressively render the remote areas hypercontractile and, consequently, crucial for global LV function;
2. Extent and severity of coronary artery disease;
3. Unfavourable anatomy for PCI;
4. Severity of LV dysfunction determined by the acute ischemic insult.

Emergent CABG has been indicated as first-choice treatment in selected patients since the early Nineties at our institution. Schematically, we now consider CABG in the following settings:

1. Left main or left main equivalent disease;
2. extensive infarction within 6-8 hours from onset, multivessel disease and critical LAD stenosis;
3. postinfarction pump failure or cardiogenic shock. The latter often ensues after 6-8 hours from the onset of ischemia and usually relates to failing remote myocardium in multivessel disease.

The vast majority of patients who undergo emergency CABG have an acutely occluded LAD and left main or three-vessel disease.

A very complex point concerns the definition of contraindications for salvage CABG. True quantification of operative risk and risk-to-benefit ratio is difficult in very high-risk surgical candidates, and valid criteria to deny surgery must be identified on an individual basis. Contraindications cannot be generalized and are often related to very advanced age, extremely poor LV function, repeated or prolonged cardiopulmonary resuscitation for arrest due to non-electrical causes (refractory pump failure), or comorbidities.

Surgical Technique

The constant phylosophy of our group has been to provide controlled reperfusion of ischemic myocardium at time of reperfusion, and complete revascularization. This distinction is important because the strategy in acute ischemia (within 6-8 hours) conceptually differs from the approach to cardiogenic shock. In the former, controlled reperfusion is primarily indicated for salvage revascularization of the infarcted area. In the latter, CABG is indicated even beyong the 6-8 hours from onset, and is performed for salvage reperfusion of the failing remote myocardium.

Since the early phase of our personal experience with emergency CABG for acute myocardial infarction [35], the surgical strategy has gradually changed. Operations are performed on cardiopulmonary bypass hypothermic with routine LV venting through the right superior pulmonary vein. Until recently, we applied mild-to-moderate systemic hypothermia (32-34 °C core temperature) and followed a modified Buckberg protocol for energy-depleted hearts, consisting of substrate-enriched (aspartate and glutamate) antegrade and retrograde cold blood cardioplegia, normothermic induction, and a 20-minute controlled reperfusion period [36]. The essential modification relates to a wider use of retrograde cardioplegia, which may prove superior after acute coronary occlusion, especially during reperfusion, in view of the probability of concomitant remote myocardial stunning [37]. As a result, maintaining doses are delivered retrograde only, avoiding interrupting the operation, the 20-minute reperfusion is performed retrogradely with the aorta clamped during construction of the proximal anastomoses, and, usually, the LAD is bypass with the internal mammary artery. If necessary, the latter is harvested after institution of cardiopulmonary bypass.

More recently, improved results have been described with on-pump beating-heart revascularization in patients with acute coronary syndromes [38-40]. Consequently, we investigated a strategy to provide controlled reperfusion, which represents the key of sophisticated cardioplegic protocols, on the beating heart. CABG is performed on full conventional cardiopulmonary bypass. The LV is vented and an intraaortic ballon pump (IABP) is routinely inserted preoperatively. Counterpulsation is maintained to provide pulsatile flow. The LAD, which is generally acutely occluded, is bypassed first. The heart is subsequently tilted and saphenous vein grafts are anastomosed to the other coronary targets. Intracoronary shunts are not used, whereas a coronary stabilizer is employed as needed. After completion of the distal anastomosis, each graft is connected proximally to the cardioplegia circuit, and controlled selective perfusion started by the perfusionist with the implementation of glutamate and asparate, for a minimum a of 20 minutes. Veins are subsequently anastomosed to the ascending aorta during a single period of side-biting clamping. Initial results with this approach have been encouraging showing a trend toward reduced perioperative myocardial damage and enzyme release. Thus, unless judged unadvisable for technical reasons, cardioplegia is now avoided, with particular emphasis on patients with ongoing heart failure and cardiogenic shock.

CONCLUSION

Summarizing, CABG has an established role in patients with poor LV function and heart failure in the chronic and acute setting. One-stage complete revascularization and controlled reperfusion are unique features of a surgical approach to myocardial ischemia, which are likely to be most benficial in the sickest patients.

REFERENCES

[1]   Favaloro, RG. Saphenous vein graft in the surgical treatment of coronary artery disease. Operative technique. *J. Thorac. Cardiovasc. Surg.,* 1969, 58, 178-85.

[2]   Nilsson, J; Algottson, L; Höglund, P; Lührs, C; Brandt, J. Early mortality in coronary bypass surgery: the EuroSCORE versus The Society of Thoracic Surgeons risk algorithm. *Ann. Thorac. Surg.,* 2004, 77, 1235-40.

[3]   Hannan, EL; Wu C; Bennett EW; et al. Risk stratification for in-hospital mortality for coronary artery bypass graft surgery. *J. Am. Coll. Cardiol.,* 2006, 47, 661-8.

[4]   Solomon, SD; Anavekar, NS; Greaves, S; Rouleau, JL; Hennekens, C; Pfeffer, MA. for the HEART Investigators. Angina pectoris prior to myocardial infarction protects against subsequent left ventricular remodeling. *J. Am. Coll. Cardiol.,* 2004, 43, 1511-4.

[5]   Dreyfus, G; Duboc, D; Blasco, A; et al. Coronary surgery can be an alternative to heart transplantation in selected patients with end-stage ischemic heart disease. *Eur. J. Cardiothorac. Surg.,* 1993, 7, 482-8.

[6]   Elefteriades, J; Edwards, R. Coronary bypass in left heart failure. *Semin. Thorac. Cardiovasc. Surg.,* 2002, 14, 125-32.

[7]   Pocar, M; Moneta, A; Grossi, A; Donatelli, F. Coronary artery bypass for heart failure in ischemic cardiomyopathy: 17-year follow-up. *Ann. Thorac. Surg.,* 2007, 83, 468-74.

[8]   Hong, H; Aksenov S; Guan, X; Fallon, JT; Waters, D; Chen, C. Remodeling of small intramyocardial coronary arteries distal to a severe epicardial coronary artery stenosis. *Arterioscler. Thromb. Vasc. Biol.,* 2002, 22, 2059-65.

[9]   Senior, R; Kaul, S; Raval, U; Lahiri, A. Impact of revascularization and myocardial viability determined by nitrate-enhanced Tc-99m sestamibi and Tl-201 imaging on mortality and functional outcome in ischemic cardiomyopathy. *J. Nucl. Cardiol.,* 2002, 9, 454-62.

[10]   Murashita, T; Makino, Y; Kamikubo, Y; Yasuda, K; Mabuchi, M; Tamaki, N. Quantitative gated myocardial perfusion single photon emission computed tomography improves the prediction of regional functional recovery in akinetic areas after coronary bypass surgery: useful tool for evaluation of myocardial viability. *J. Thorac. Cardiovasc. Surg.,* 2003, 126, 1328-34.

[11]   Wu, YW; Tadamura, E; Yamamuro, M; et al. Comparison of contrast-enhanced MRI with (18)F-FDG PET/201Tl SPECT in dysfunctional myocardium: relation to early functional outcome after surgical revascularization in chronic ischemic heart disease. *J. Nucl. Med.* 2007, 48, 1096-103. Erratum in: *J. Nucl. Med.,* 2007, 48, 1789.

[12]   Samady, H; Liu, YH; Choi, CJ; et al. Electromechanical mapping for detecting myocardial viability and ischemia in patients with severe ischemic cardiomyopathy. *Am. J. Cardiol.,* 2003, 91, 807-11.

[13]   Ogawa, M; Doi, K; Fukumoto, A; Yaku, H. Reverse-remodeling after coronary artery bypass grafting in ischemic cardiomyopathy: assessment of myocardial viability by delayed-enhanced magnetic resonance imaging can help cardiac surgeons. *Interact Cardiovasc. Thorac. Surg.,* 2007, 6, 673-5.

[14]   Rizzello, V; Poldermans, D; Boersma, E; et al. Opposite patterns of left ventricular remodeling after coronary revascularization in patients with ischemic cardiomyopathy. Role of myocardial viability. *Circulation.,* 2004, 110, 2383-8.

[15]   Meharwal, ZS; Mishra, YK; Kohli, V; Bapna, R; Singh, S; Trehan, N. Off-pump multivessel coronary artery surgery in high-risk patients. *Ann. Thorac. Surg.,* 2002, 74, S1353-7.

[16] Balacumaraswami, L; Abu-Omar, Y; Selvanayagam, J; Pigott, D; Taggart, DP. The effects of on-pump and off-pump coronary artery bypass grafting on intraoperative graft flow in arterial and venous conduits defined by a flow-pressure ratio. *J. Thorac. Cardiovasc.*, Surg 2008, 135, 533-9.

[17] Rosenkranz, ER; Okamoto, F; Buckberg, GD; Robertson, JM; Vinten-Johansen, J; Bugyi, HI. Safety of prolonged aortic clamping with blood cardioplegia. III. Aspartate enrichment of glutamate-blood cardioplegia in energy-depleted hearts after ischemic and reperfusion injury. *J. Thorac. Cardiovasc. Surg.*, 1986, 91, 428-35.

[18] Skalidis, EL; Parthenakis, FI; Patrianakos, AP; Hamilos, MI; Vradas, PE. Regional coronary flow and contractile reserve in patients with idiopathic dilated cardiomyopathy. *J. Am. Coll. Cardiol.*, 2004, 44, 2027-32.

[19] Jegaden, O; Bontemps, L; de Gevigney, G; et al. Does the extended use of arterial grafts compromise the myocardial recovery after coronary artery bypass grafting in left ventricular dysfunction? *Eur. J. Cardiothorac. Surg.*, 1998, 14, 353-9.

[20] Gaudiani, VA; Castro, LJ; Fisher, AL. Biventricular pacing during cardiac operations. *Heart Surg. Forum.*, 2003, 6, E126-8.

[21] Tolis, GA; Jr; Korkolis, DP; Kopf, GS; Elefteriades, JA. Revascularization alone (without mitral valve repair) suffices in patients with advanced ischemic cardiomyopathy and mild-to-moderate mitral regurgitation. *Ann. Thorac. Surg.*, 2002, 74, 1476-881.

[22] Diodato, MD; Moon,; Pasque, MK; et al. Repair of ischemic mitral regurgitation does not increase mortality or improve long-term survival in patients undergoing coronary artery revascularization, a propensity analysis. *Ann. Thorac. Surg.*, 2004, 78, 794-9.

[23] Glower, DD; Tuttle, RH; Shaw, LK; Orozco, RE; Rankin, JS. Patient survival characteristics after routine mitral valve repair for ischemic mitral regurgitation. *J. Thorac. Cardiovasc. Surg.*, 2005, 129, 860-8.

[24] Kang, DH; Kim, MJ; Kang, SJ; et al. Mitral valve repair versus revascularization alone in the treatment of ischemic mitral regurgitation. *Circulation.*, 2006, 114(1 Suppl), I499-503.

[25] Mihaljevic, T; Lam, BK; Rajeswaran, J; et al. Impact of mitral valve annuloplasty combined with revascularization in patients with functional ischemic mitral regurgitation. *J. Am. Coll. Cardiol.*, 2007, 49, 2191-201.

[26] Grigioni, F; Enriquez-Sarano, M; Zehr, KJ; Bailey, KR; Taji, AJ. Ischemic mitral regurgitation: long-term outcome and prognostic

implications with quantitative Doppler assessment. *Circulation.*, 2001, 103, 1759-64.

[27] Vaskelyte, J; Stoskute, N; Kinduris, S; Ereminiene, E. Coronary artery bypass grafting in patients with severe left ventricular dysfunction: predictive significance of left ventricular diastolic filling pattern. *Eur. J. Echocardiogr.*, 2001, 2, 62-7.

[28] Møller, JE; Hillis, GS; Oh, JK; et al. Left atrial volume. A powerful predictor of survival after acute myocardial infarction. *Circulation.*, 2003, 107, 2207-12.

[29] Favaloro, RG; Effler, DB; Cheanvechai, C; Quint, RA; Sones, FM; Jr. Acute coronary insufficieincy (impending myocardial infarction and myocardial infarction): surgical treatment by the saphenous vein graft technique. *Am. J. Cardiol.*, 1971, 28, 598-607.

[30] Yusuf, S; Sleight, P; Held, P; et al. Routine medical management of acute myocardial infarction. Lessond from overviews of recent randomized control trials. *Circulation.*, 1990, 82 (Suppl. II):II-117-II-134.

[31] Koshal, A; Beanlands, DS; Davies, RA; et al. Urgent surgical reperfusion in acute evolving myocardial infarction. *Circulation.*, 1988, 78 (Suppl. I), I-171-I-178.

[32] Barner, HB; Lea, JW, IV; Naunheim, KS; et al. Emergency coronary bypass not associated with preoperative cardiogenic shock in failed angioplasty, after thrombolysis, and for acute myocardial infarction. *Circulation.*, 1989, 79 (Suppl. I), I-152-I-159.

[33] Hochman, JS; Sleeper, LA; Webb, JG; et al. Early revascularization and long-term survival in cardiogenic shock complicating acute myocardial infarction. *JAMA.*, 2006, 295, 2511-5.

[34] White, HD; Assmann, SF; Sanborn, TA; et al. Comparison of percutaneous coronary intervention and coronary artery bypass grafting after acute myocardial infarction complicated by cardiogenic shock, results from the Should We Emergently Revascularize Occluded Coronaries for Cardiogenic Shock (SHOCK) trial. *Circulation.*, 2005, 112, 1992-2001.

[35] Donatelli, F; Benussi, S; Triggiani, M; et al. Surgical treatment for life-threatening acute myocardial infarction: a prospective protocol. *Eur. J. Cardio-Thorac. Surg.*, 1997, 11, 228-33.

[36] Donatelli, F; Pocar, M; Grossi, A. Acute myocardial infarction and cardiogenic shock. In: Beyersdorf F, editor. Ischemia-reperfusion injury in cardiac surgery. *Georgetown: Landes Bioscience,* 2001, 196-202.

[37] Haan, C; Hazar, HL; Bernard, S; et al. Superiority of retrograde cardioplegia after acute coronary occlusion. *Ann. Thorac. Surg.,* 1991, 51, 408-12.

[38] Edgerton, JR; Herbert, MA; Jones, KK; et al. On-pump beating heart surgery offers an alternative for unstable patients undergoing coronary artery bypass grafting. *Heart Surg. Forum.,* 2004, 7, 8-15.

[39] Izumi, Y; Magishi, K; H Ishikawa, N; Kimura, F. On-pump beating-heart coronary artery bypass grafting for acute myocardial infarction. *Ann. Thorac. Surg.,* 2006, 81, 573-6.

[40] Rastan, AJ; Eckenstein, JI; Hentschel, B; et al. Emergency coronary artery bypass graft surgery for acute coronary syndrome: beating heart versus conventional cardioplegic cardiac arrest strategies. *Circulation.,* 2006, 114, I477-85.

INDEX

D

H

I